DELECTABLY WHOLE

MEC-LYNN LEE

DELECTABLY WHOLE

Gluten-Free | Dairy-Free | Refined Sugar-Free
Suitable for those on a Paleo, FODMAP or Histamine-friendly diet

Gold-Crested
Press

CONTENTS

MY STORY	7
PANTRY STAPLES	11
EXPLORING THE WORLD OF ALTERNATIVE BAKING	12
BISCUITS	16
Sweet Potato Biscuits	19
Anzac Biscuits	20
Almond Crescents	23
Macadamia Cranberry Biscuits	24
Jam Drop Biscuits	27
Gingernut Biscuits	28
Chocolate Chip Biscuits	31
CAKES & MUFFINS	32
Blood Orange Poppy Seed Muffins	35
Breakfast Muffins to Boost	36
Double Chocolate Banana Zucchini Blueberry Muffins	39
Lemon Yoghurt Tea Cake	40
Carrot Cake	43
Lamingtons with Raspberry Jam	44
SLICES & TARTS	48
Twist On The Twix	51
Strawberry Jelly Slices	52
Blueberry Frangipane Tart	57
Pecan Tart	58
Lemon Curd Tartlets	61
Baked Oat Granola Bars	62
SWEET TREATS	64
Cinnamon Doughnuts	67
Banana Pancakes	68
Fudgy Chocolate Brownies	71
Tiramisu	72
Sticky Banana Puddings with Caramel Sauce	77
Chocolate Self-Saucing Puddings	78
Apple Crumble	81

BREADS, PASTRY & CEREALS	82
Gluten-Free Flour Blend – Option 1	84
Gluten-Free Flour Blend – Option 2	84
Slice and Tart Base – Option 1	85
Slice and Tart Base – Option 2	86
Slice and Tart Base – Option 3	87
Gluten & Yeast-Free Sandwich Bread Loaf	89
Pita Flatbread Wraps	90
Gluten-Free Bagels	93
Scones	94
Gluten-Free Pizza Bases	97
Muesli	99
CONDIMENTS	100
Blueberry Jam	103
Caramel Sauce	104
Herb Macadamia Pesto	107
Dad's Ginger Spring Onion Sauce	108
SAVOURY SENSATIONS	110
Baked Maple Lemon-Glazed Chicken	113
Salmon Sweet Potato Fritters	114
Pork & Chicken Pot Sticker Dumplings	117
Creamy Thai Chicken Curry	121
Frittata	122
Pork & Turkey Sausage Rolls	125
Roast Chicken Rice Feast	129
Crackling Roast Pork Belly	130
Vegetable Soup	134
Baked Garlic & Rosemary Sweet Potato Chips	137
ASIAN DELICACIES	138
Kaya	141
Pandan Sponge Cake	142
Pineapple Tarts	147
Baked Egg Tarts	148
REFERENCES	152
GRATITUDE	153

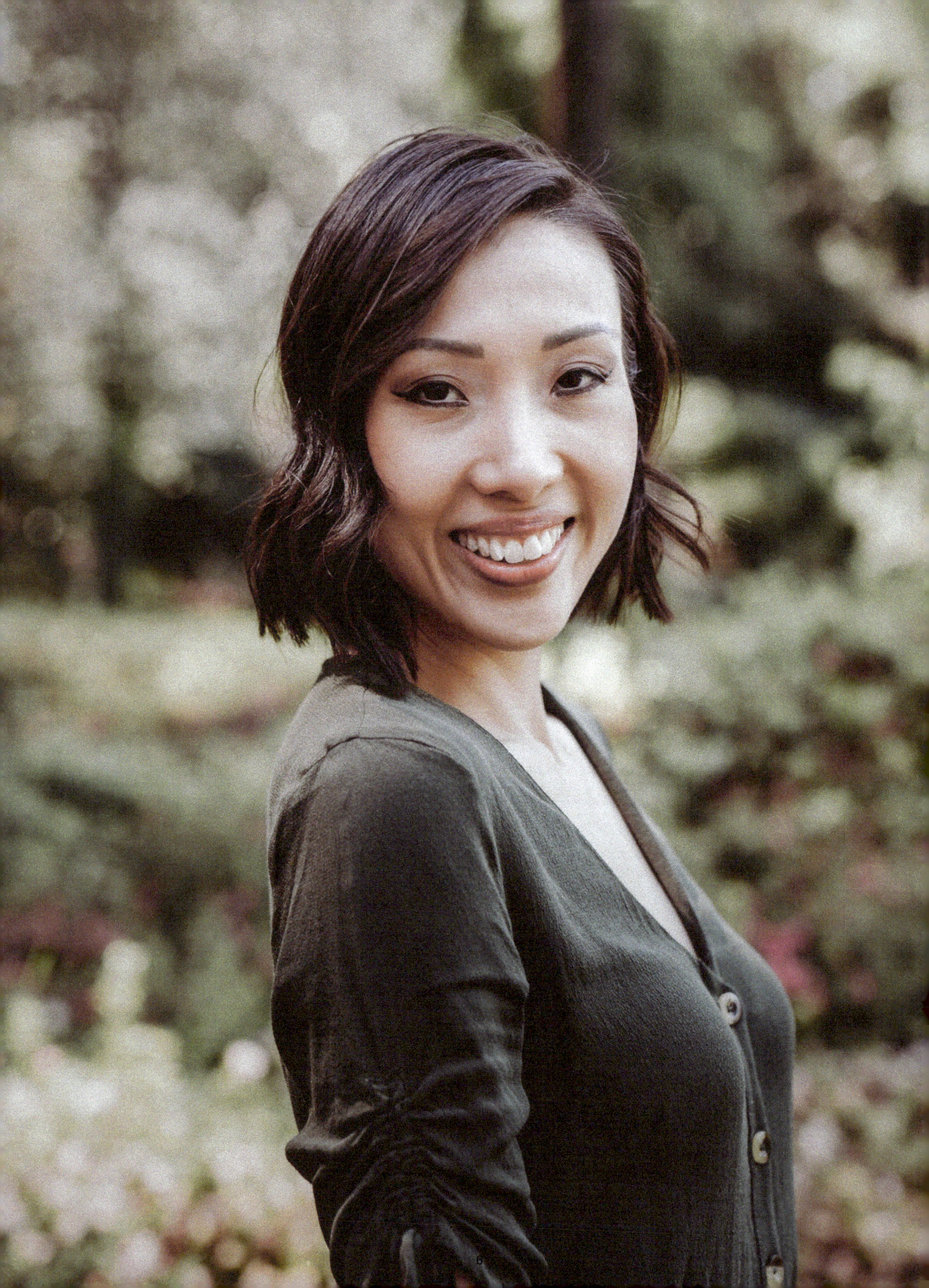

MY STORY

Hello, beautiful readers and aspiring cooks! My name is Mec-Lynn, and it is an absolute joy to be able to share my journey of navigating through the past two decades, in the hope that it will inspire, encourage and ignite hope in your life or the lives of your friends and family.

Some of you may have been struggling with food intolerances for most of your life, or perhaps you have only just recently discovered these health issues. Maybe you know someone who is facing challenging health battles. Or making some lifestyle changes to live your best healthy life possible is something you want or need to do.

Whatever the reason, I am here to encourage those who feel they have been missing out on great tasting, healthy foods - there is hope! I invite you to immerse yourself in these extraordinary recipes and begin a journey of learning to use fresh and wholesome ingredients, some of which you may have never used or tasted before, and to get creative in the kitchen. As my wise late grandfather used to say — "One must never stop learning!"

WHERE IT ALL STARTED...

My family and I migrated to Melbourne, Australia from Kuala Lumpur, Malaysia when I was four days shy of turning ten years old. I recall how quickly I needed to adapt to the Australian culture and way of life as a new migrant. Today, I am so proud to call Australia my home.

I had been a healthy, robust child; energetic, carefree, cheeky, inquisitive in nature and an adventure-seeker. A few months after turning twelve, I experienced severe gastroenteritis which was the catalyst for many health issues that followed. For the next twenty years, I was in and out of GPs, specialist offices, hospitals, naturopaths, and speech pathologists. I underwent multiple gastroscopies, colonoscopies, MRIs, blood tests – the list goes on. I was practically a walking medical dictionary and became quite knowledgeable on everything to do with the gut, digestion, swallowing, FODMAPS, histamine levels, different foods and their nutritional properties, the power of the gut-brain relationship and everything in between. There were periods where I would feel amazing and invincible, only to come back full circle and sometimes struggle just to get out of bed in the morning.

My health was manageable up until the time I went on a mission's trip in July 2017, where new and debilitating symptoms emerged, sending my body on a rollercoaster ride that I could not get off. The next three years were the most crucial time for my healing journey, where I began seeing an Integrated Gut Specialist for a year and a half. He helped create awareness of some of the issues happening in my body and addressed them with natural supplements. There were many possible theories relating to my symptoms but till today, I still do not have a clear diagnosis.

This was a reset moment for me. I began intently researching what foods were appropriate in helping my body to heal and switched to organic produce. I eliminated all gluten, dairy, refined sugar, and heavy spices from my diet. I stopped eating out and started to cook all of my meals, which are made with wholesome, quality ingredients.

I was also introduced to ASEA in June 2019, where I have been drinking its Redox Cell Signalling water and applying the Renu28 Gel on problematic areas, both of which have helped me tremendously (please see footnote* for more information and links).

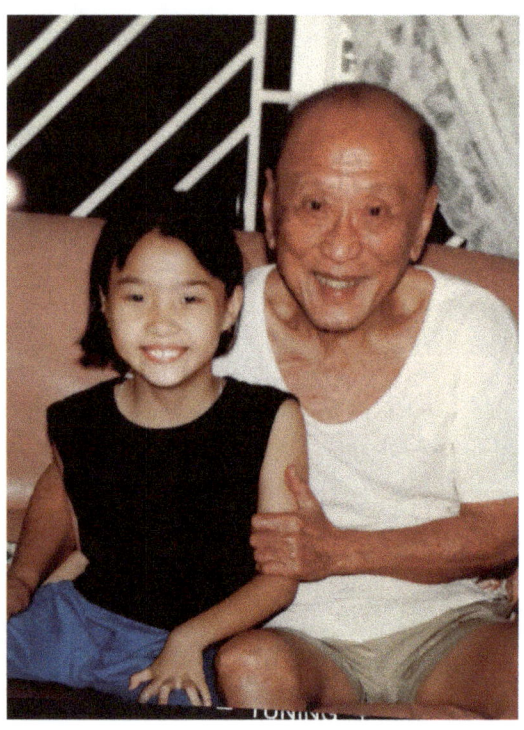
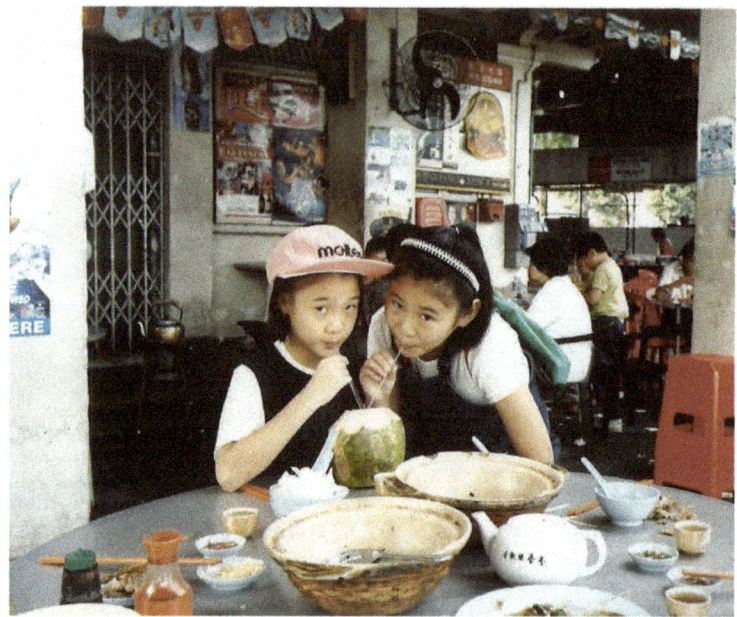

In addition to the physical aspects of healing, I decided to take steps in ensuring a more holistic approach to my overall wellbeing, by seeing a psychologist to help with the mental and emotional impact my illness has had over the years. I sought help to turn my focus and attention from the negativity, frustration, helplessness and confusion caused by my illness, to pursuing greater intimacy with God and strengthening my spiritual life.

It is challenging to summarise my thirty years of life and the pilgrimage I have been on in a few paragraphs, but it gives you a brief snapshot of where I am at today. By the grace and goodness of God, I am on the road to recovery and I would not be where I am today without Him.

WHERE PASSION FOR FOOD GREW...
My love and passion for all things related to food began as a child growing up in Malaysia. I would often shadow my grandmother and mother while they cooked in the kitchen, trying to procrastinate doing my homework. The glorious smells and tantalising flavours always enticed and excited me. I relished the opportunity to watch them cook and have a go myself. Sometimes, they would shoo me away to get my homework done or because I wasn't old enough, which made me all the more determined to learn how to cook from a very young age. My grandparents would often bring home sumptuous savoury and sweet treats from the street stalls for our afternoon snacks after school. On many weekends, my parents would take us out to eat local and culturally diverse fare, and every special occasion was a good reason to feast!

I looked forward to our yearly Chinese New Year celebrations when we would drive down to Johor Bahru to stay with our grandparents and extended family. My grandparents' hospitality and generosity always extended in leaps and bounds, as feeding us was a huge love language for them.

During my teenage years, I loved eating all kinds of desserts and aspired to be a pastry chef. I would seize any opportunity to bake - for special occasions or just for the fun of it. Family and friends were always eager to try my baked treats and

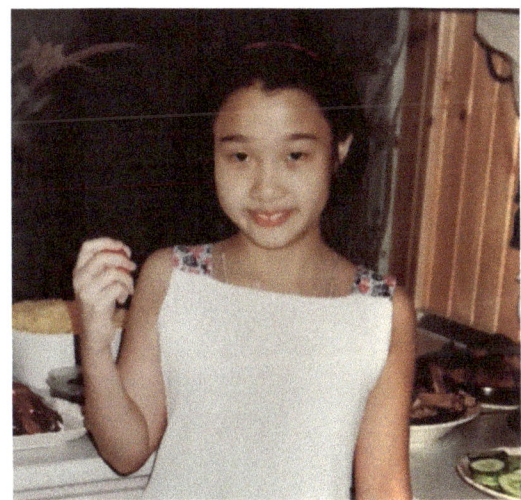
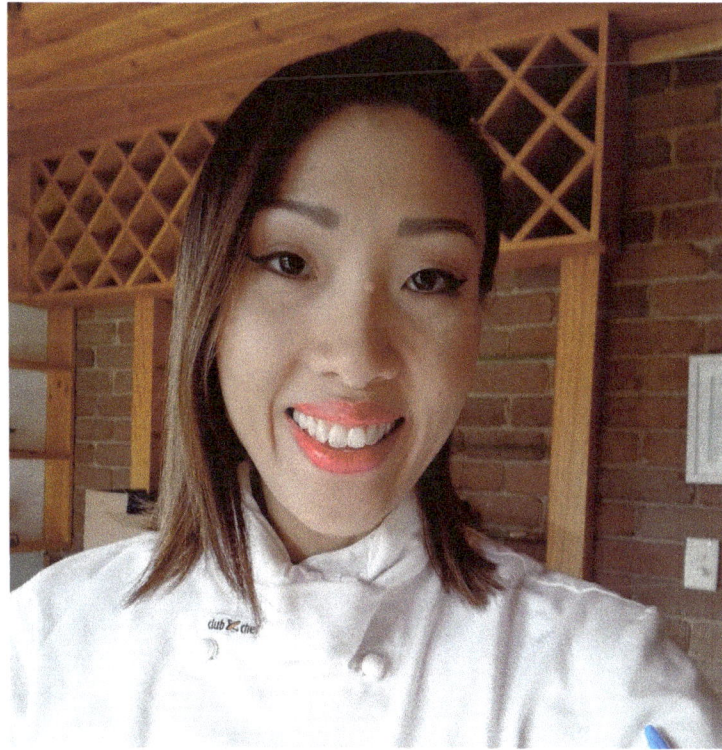

seemed to enjoy them very much! This passion led me to gain a degree in culinary management, where I learnt a lot about business management in the culinary world.

Being Malaysian Chinese – food is everything and it plays such an integral role in bringing family and loved ones together. We live to eat! I finally decided I was not going to be robbed of my enjoyment of food because of my illness. But what was a girl to do when all she had ever known was to bake with wheat flour, butter and sugar? Thus began months and years of intense research into the world of alternative ingredients and experimental baking; trying to create the perfect chocolate chip cookie or a brownie that closely resembled its sugar and gluten-loaded counterpart. What I discovered to my surprise, was that the healthy version tasted way better than what you would buy at the store! What's even better, most recipes only require a bowl and a whisk or wooden spoon (no stand mixer required) and the different flour options are endless! The more I baked, cooked and shared, the more people encouraged me to write my very own cookbook. How could I keep these recipes to myself? I had to share it with the world.

That is how 'Delectably Whole' was born. By sharing my recipes with you, I hope to empower you with the knowledge so you can create timeless recipes of your own, tailored to your health needs, without compromising on flavour! My earnest desire is that you will fall in love with food again and that you will rediscover the joy of eating your favourite dish, knowing you are feeding your body with the good stuff. When we care and look after our bodies, we become an inspiration for others to do the same! My healing journey continues even as I write this book. I look positively into the future, believing that the best is yet to come. So, come along with me in becoming the best, healthiest version that you can be, and most importantly, have fun creating in the kitchen!

Much love,
Mec-Lynn xoxo

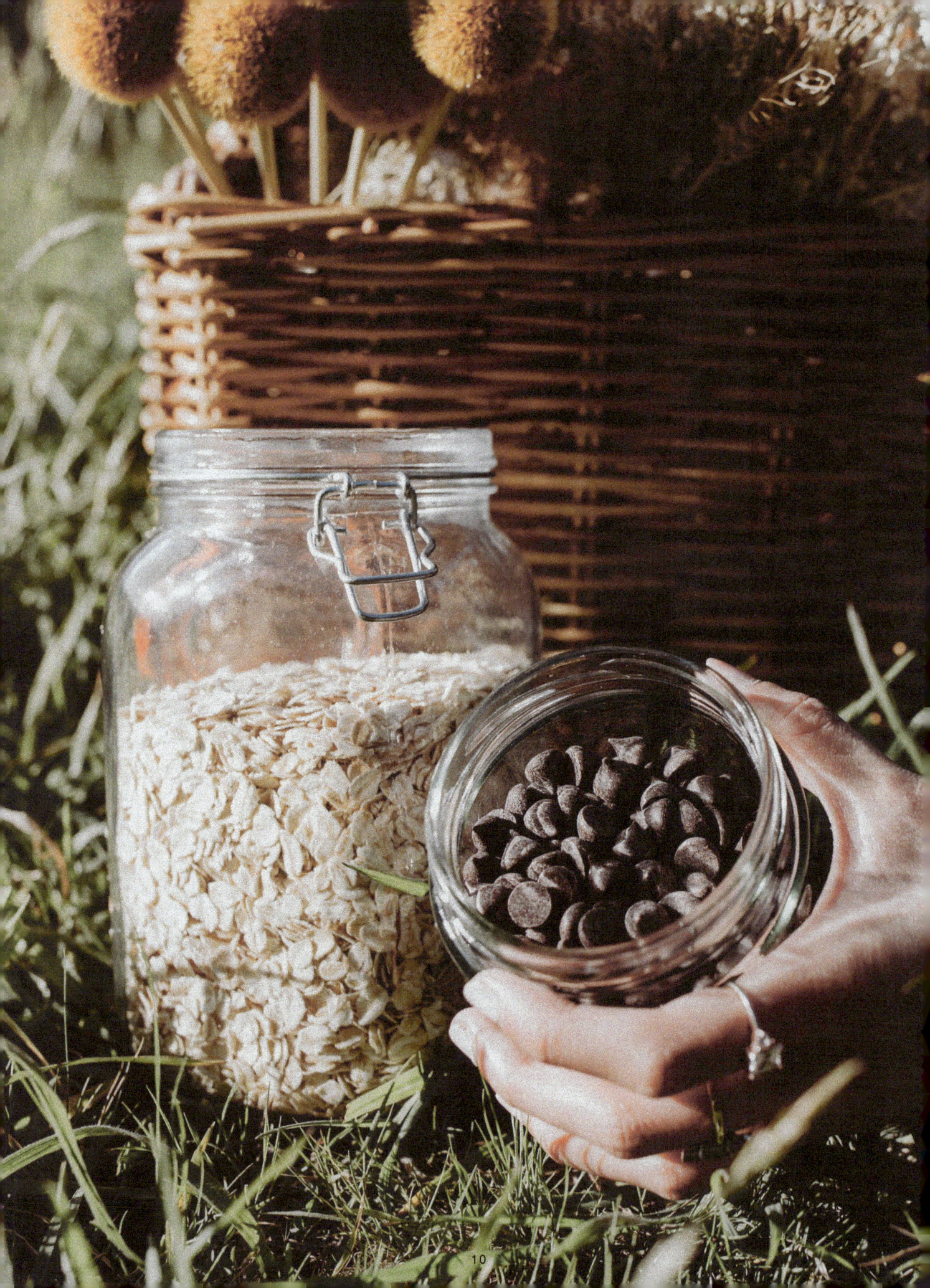

PANTRY STAPLES

FLOURS & STARCHES

Blanched almond flour
Organic millet flour
Organic sorghum flour
Organic teff flour
Organic tiger nut flour
Organic hemp flour
Organic desiccated coconut (no preservatives and sulphites)
Organic brown rice flour
Glutinous rice flour
Organic green banana flour
Organic tapioca starch (no preservatives and sulphites)
Organic arrowroot starch (no preservatives and sulphites)
Organic potato starch (no preservatives and sulphites)
Organic cassava flour
Organic quinoa flour
Organic oat flour (blended rolled oats)

OILS & BUTTERS

Organic extra virgin coconut oil
Garlic-infused olive oil
Organic coconut butter
Organic cacao butter
Organic almond butter
Vegan butter
Organic sunflower seed butter
Organic unhulled tahini

NATURAL SWEETENERS

Pure organic unsweetened applesauce (store-bought or make your own)
Organic unrefined coconut sugar
Organic raw coconut flower nectar sugar
Organic pure maple sugar
Pure maple syrup (not the nasty flavoured stuff)

CHOCOLATE

Dark chocolate chips, 70% preferred
Dark baking chocolate, 70% preferred
Organic cacao powder

OTHER - DRY

Organic golden flaxseed meal
Organic coconut flour (no preservatives and sulphites)
Organic coconut powder
Organic rolled oats
Gluten-free baking soda
Gluten-free baking powder
Dried cranberries (apple juice-sweetened)
Assorted nuts and low-histamine seeds – almonds, pecans, macadamias, brazil nuts, pepitas and sunflower seeds
Pink Himalayan sea salt
Agar-agar flakes

OTHER - WET

Pure vanilla extract (none of that imitation essence)
Apple cider vinegar (with the mother)
Unsweetened plant-based milk (e.g.: almond milk, rice milk, soy milk, oat milk)
Unsweetened coconut yoghurt
Organic 100% coconut cream & coconut milk

FOOTNOTES

There isn't any baking chocolate readily available in stores that do not contain refined sugars, so I have relied on ones that use organic raw sugar instead. However, I have recently discovered Solomons Gold chocolates which only contain pure coconut nectar as the sweetener of choice. They also sell dark chocolate pieces for baking purposes online.

Recommended brands include: Solomons Gold, Green & Blacks Organic 70% and 85%, Pico Super Dark 85%, Magic Chocolate 47%-84%, Pana Organic Mylk and Tonantzin Aztec Artisan Chocolate 60% and 80%

EXPLORING THE WORLD OF ALTERNATIVE BAKING

Some of the ingredients used in these recipes such as chocolate, cacao powder, bananas, dried fruit, yoghurt or tomatoes are considered histamine-inducing. However, I have found that when used minimally and not eaten accumulatively, I have not reacted negatively to them. As always, serving quantities, using your discretion and listening to your body are all crucial in navigating your health journey.

AGAR-AGAR FLAKES, otherwise known as 'Kanten' in Japanese, is the plant-based equivalent to gelatin. It is derived by extracting the carbohydrates from the red algae seaweed and is often found in the form of flakes, powder, strands or a bar. Agar-agar is used to thicken and stabilise foods but requires being heated over the stove to dissolve and set, as opposed to gelatin which can be dissolved in water and added to foods. It provides a much firmer and less creamy texture, but this can also depend on the quantity used. Although agar-agar powder is an exact substitute to gelatin powder, you will need more agar flakes, as 1 tablespoon of agar flakes is equivalent to 1 teaspoon of agar powder. For foods with higher acidity like those containing citrus, more agar-agar needs to be added to the cooking process for them to set. While agar-agar is tasteless and odourless, it is a wonderful source of calcium, fibre, iron, manganese and folate.

ALMOND BUTTER (or any other nut or seed butter you prefer) is a great ingredient to add to cookies, muffins, brownies, bliss balls or as the foundation for making caramel, as it provides a rich, nutty, chewy texture and binds well. It is also packed with heart-healthy fats and fibre, vitamins, minerals and antioxidants, supports brain function and controls blood sugar levels. Similarly to almond flour or meal, it is considered moderate FODMAP as the phytic acid in almonds can irritate the gut. Therefore, I try to use smaller amounts and blend with other gluten-free flours in my recipes (unless the recipe is primarily almond-based).

APPLE CIDER VINEGAR (WITH THE MOTHER) is pure magic when added to baked goods. It is perfect when combined with plant-based milk for making dairy-free buttermilk to give muffins and cakes a light, moist texture. It also reacts chemically with baking soda to help give rise and aeration, and can give tart pastries that extra flakiness. Best of all, it has so many health benefits including lowering blood pressure and cholesterol, aiding in weight loss, improving skin health, detoxification and gut health.

BLANCHED ALMOND FLOUR is very similar to almond meal, just without the almond skin. It is much finer in texture and is perfect for use as an addition to other flours in gluten-free baked goods, as the fat content creates a more tender and moist texture while the almonds lend a subtle sweetness and aroma. Although almond flour is full of health benefits such as fibre, iron, calcium, manganese, vitamin E, magnesium and potassium, it is considered moderate FODMAP as the phytic acid can irritate the gut. Therefore, I try to use smaller amounts and blend with other gluten-free flours in my recipes (unless the recipe is primarily almond-based).

CACAO POWDER is essentially pure chocolate obtained from cold-pressing unroasted cacao beans, thus preserving its nutritional value. This is different to cocoa powder or Dutch-processed cocoa powder, which is made by roasting cacao beans at high temperatures and processing it with alkali to reduce the acidity content. Cacao powder is full of powerful antioxidants, magnesium and sulfur; promoting heart health, balancing cholesterol levels and lowering blood pressure. Due to its raw state, it is bitterer than cocoa powder, so be sure to increase the quantity of natural sweeteners to balance out the bitterness. It is perfect to use in anything requiring a chocolatey flavour, as well as combining it with cacao butter to make pure chocolate.

COCONUT BUTTER is simply dried coconut grounded up into a smooth butter, with all the fibre included. It contains fibre and iron, aids in weight loss, boosts immunity and is full of healthy fats. Coconut butter is perfect for making icing, drizzling on baked treats or when making fudge. It can also be a good substitute for different kinds of nut butter for those who are allergic to nuts.

COCONUT FLOWER NECTAR SUGAR derives from dehydrating the sap or nectar tapped from the stems of the coconut blossoms at the top of the coconut tree. It is mildly sweet and usually appears in a larger crystalised form. It is low GI, rich in nutrients and vitamins and contains 17 amino acids. This sugar is perfect for sprinkling on cookies, doughnuts or processed more finely to be used in baking.

COCONUT OIL is a key ingredient in many alternative baking recipes as it is dairy-free, natural and so versatile. It does not contain harmful toxins found in other hydrogenated cooking oils, prevents heart disease and high blood pressure, improves energy and digestion and provides a pleasant coconut flavour to baked goods. You can use it in its solid state or melted.

COCONUT SUGAR is made from boiling and dehydrating the sap or nectar collected from coconut palm trees. It is an unrefined natural sweetener and has similar characteristics to brown sugar. Although coconut sugar is low GI and contains trace amounts of vitamins and minerals, it is still sugar and moderately high in fructose. Thus, it is not used in large quantities in my recipes.

GLUTINOUS RICE FLOUR can also be referred to as sweet rice flour or sticky rice flour. Ironically, as the name suggests, it actually does not contain any gluten but is a wonderful starch binder in baked goods due to its sticky chewy texture when heated or cooked. It is made by milling long or short grain sweet white rice, both types suitable for different baking purposes. Glutinous rice flour is most commonly used in Asian sweet and savoury dishes such as Japanese mochi, dumplings and fried dough balls with sweet filling. This flour should not be used in replacement of rice flour, as they cook differently and produce very different results. I have added glutinous rice flour to one of my gluten-free flour blends, as it works well with other starches and whole grain flours in providing structure and aiding in texture, especially when avoiding additional ingredients like xantham gum.

MAPLE SUGAR is made by boiling maple syrup to a certain point before it begins to caramelise and harden, turning into granulated sugar. It is a great unrefined natural sweetener to use instead of maple syrup if the recipe calls for less liquid and a dryer crumb, or to maintain a lighter colour in the final product, compared to using coconut sugar. It is also a good substitute for icing sugar, when processed to a fine powder.

MAPLE SYRUP (PURE) is obtained from boiling the sap collected from sugar maple trees and can come in Grade A (lighter) or Grade B (darker) versions. It is packed with antioxidants, is low GI, improves digestion and is full of vitamins and minerals such as manganese, zinc, potassium and calcium. Most of my recipes heavily rely on maple syrup as the natural sweetener of choice, especially as it is low fructose compared to honey.

ORGANIC ARROWROOT STARCH (no preservatives and sulphites) was first cultivated in the Caribbean Islands and comes from the tubers of a tropical American herb or the entire vegetable plant itself and was known for its healing properties in the Central American region. It is often used interchangeably with tapioca starch or potato starch in thickening foods, however, it is also one of the easiest starches to digest, especially for those with sensitive digestive systems. Arrowroot has incredible anti-inflammatory properties and helps to alleviate digestive problems, boosts immunity, fights foodborne pathogens and soothes pain. This starch is great in desserts and baking as it provides body and structure to the baked goods.

ORGANIC BROWN RICE FLOUR is obtained from grinding wholegrain brown rice in its entirety, thus keeping all the nutritional properties compared to that of white rice flour. It contains a higher fibre content, iron, phosphorus and potassium. It has a mild nutty flavour profile and is a great addition to your gluten-free flour mix, as it is considered a 'heavy' flour.

ORGANIC CACAO BUTTER is the vegetable fat extracted from cold-pressing unroasted cacao beans and provides the rich aroma of dark chocolate.

ORGANIC CACAO POWDER combined with cacao butter, vanilla and a sweetener of choice makes for glorious tasting chocolate products such as chocolate bark, chocolate icing and many other chocolate-flavoured things.

ORGANIC CASSAVA FLOUR is made through the process of grating, drying and grounding the cassava or yuca root, native to South America. Cassava contains good sources of minerals like copper and potassium, folate, manganese and thiamine as well as being high in vitamin C which aids in healthier skin, gums, teeth and fights free-radical damage. It is also low in fat, sugar and calories and acts as a prebiotic fibre which is both anti-inflammatory and aids in digestion. It is not the same as tapioca starch, as tapioca starch is extracted from the root through the process of squeezing the pulp, leaving behind the starchy liquid and evaporating its water content. Popular in paleo baking, it is grain-free, nut-free and gluten-free with a similar taste and texture to wheat. Just reduce the volume by a quarter when measuring in cups as a substitute for gluten flour.

ORGANIC COCONUT FLOUR (no preservatives and sulphites) is the by-product of drying and grinding coconut meat once the coconut milk is extracted. It is packed with protein, fibre, manganese and fat and is relatively low in carbohydrates. Although wonderful to use in baked goods, it can be quite tricky to bake with coconut flour due to its high absorbency of liquids, which tends to lend to a dryer end result. So, a little goes a long way! Alternatively, more eggs and liquid need to be added if you are predominantly using coconut flour in the recipe. This will alter the cooking times, structure and texture of the baked goods.

ORGANIC COCONUT POWDER is obtained from dehydrating coconut milk and adding tapioca with a small amount of natural thickeners. It is perfect to use as a substitute for icing sugar when mixed with blended maple sugar or can be returned to a coconut milk and cream consistency by dissolving it in hot water. You can add it to smoothies, savoury dishes or anything that you would use coconut milk in. Packed full of good healthy MCT fats, it also packs in all the vitamins and minerals as mentioned earlier.

ORGANIC DESICCATED COCONUT (no preservatives and sulphites) is made by drying dehusked coconuts and finely cutting them to achieve that shredded delicate consistency. Again, it is packed full of nutrients as found in its other forms and gives baked treats a chewy, moist texture with a pleasant coconut flavour. It is perfect to use in bliss balls, slices, cookies and cakes. Be sure to buy organic 100% unadulterated coconut as many commercially sold desiccated coconut products contain added preservatives which means sulphites are present.

ORGANIC GOLDEN FLAXSEED MEAL is made by grinding flaxseeds to a fine consistency. It is lighter in colour than the brown flaxseeds but equally as nutritious. Flaxseeds are packed with fibre, protein, essential omega-3 fatty acids and a host of other vitamins and minerals. Ground flaxseeds are also easier to digest and they are wonderful to add to cakes, muffins, cookies, bliss balls, bread or anything, really! They are a great egg replacer when mixed with liquid, or a substitute for chia seeds or xantham gum. They work beautifully to bind and add structure to baked goods while providing a great nutty flavour.

ORGANIC GREEN BANANA FLOUR is flour obtained from drying and grounding green bananas. Very popular in Jamaica and Africa as a wheat substitute, green banana flour is increasingly becoming well known in the gluten-free world of baking due to its gut health benefits. It is considered a resistant starch, in that it does not break down into sugars easily, thus helping with blood sugar levels, pH levels, forming good bacteria in the gut and protecting cells from damage. When cooked, it provides an earthy banana flavour and a texture similar to lighter wheat flours, pairing very well to chocolate. Like cassava flour, be sure to reduce the volume by a quarter when measuring in cups as a substitute for gluten flour.

ORGANIC HEMP FLOUR is made by grinding hemp seeds to a fine powder. Known as a superfood as well as a 'complete protein', it contains all 9 essential amino acids, omega fatty acids, anti-inflammatory properties, Vitamin D and B, Iron, Zinc, Magnesium and Calcium. This makes it for a wonderful addition to baked goods, especially in cookies, cakes, muffins and bread, providing a beautiful nutty flavour and aroma.

ORGANIC MILLET FLOUR is considered an ancient grain (although is technically a seed) that originated from Africa and has become a world-wide staple, popular in African and Indian dishes. It is made by milling the millet seeds into a fine flour. With its alkaline properties and mild sweet flavour, it is packed with nutrients including insoluble fibre, antioxidants, magnesium, iron and phosphorus. Millet flour is perfect as an addition to other gluten-free flours and lends a melt-in-your-mouth texture to cakes, muffins and cookies. It also acts as a great binder in foods as it absorbs liquid and thickens.

ORGANIC POTATO STARCH (no preservatives and sulphites) is extracted from potatoes and is most commonly used as a substitute for cornflour or arrowroot starches in thickening recipes and baked goods. It is different from potato flour, as potato flour is drying and grinding whole potatoes, thus having a stronger flavour of the potato. While potatoes themselves contain good sources of vitamins and minerals, the starch content does not equally carry this nutritional profile. However, potato starch does help with blood sugar levels, is considered a resistant starch thus acting as a great prebiotic for the bacteria in your gut and works well as part of a gluten-free flour blend. It is important to buy non-GMO potato starch.

ORGANIC QUINOA FLOUR is a superfood seed, native to Peru and Bolivia but has now become a worldwide staple. It is nutrient-rich and boasts being a complete protein, containing all 9 essential amino acids. It is also packed full of phosphorus, manganese, fibre and plenty of vitamins and minerals. With a light nutty flavour and aroma, it is perfect as an addition to other gluten-free flours in all baked goods. It is best to toast the flour for 5-10 minutes in a pan before adding to your batter, as this helps remove the slight bitterness that may infuse in your baking.

ORGANIC ROLLED OATS (uncontaminated) are naturally gluten-free as they are derived from hulled oat grains, so it is usually tolerated by gluten-intolerant people. However, if you are wanting to be extra careful, look for packaging that specifically states 'Gluten-Free'. Oats are a wonderful source of beta-glucan fibre, protein, vitamins, minerals and antioxidants such as manganese, phosphorus, thiamine and magnesium as well as being low GI, keeping you sustained and fuller for longer. Rolled oats are perfect in creating chewy texture with a nutty flavour in biscuits and granola bars or used in muesli. They can also be processed to make oat flour which is great when paired with other gluten-free flours in baked goods, providing moisture, density and structure to baked goods.

ORGANIC SORGHUM FLOUR is grounded flour made from the ancient wholegrain Sorghum, originating in Africa and Australia thousands of years ago. It is mildly sweet and softly textured, packed with iron, B vitamins, protein, antioxidants, dietary fibre, is anti-inflammatory and lowers blood sugar levels. Considered a 'heavy flour', it is best used in combination with other lighter gluten-free flours and starches.

ORGANIC TAPIOCA STARCH (no preservatives and sulphites) comes from the cassava root and is typically used in place of cornflour to thicken foods and sauces. Although not high in nutritional properties, apart from being a low-calorie sugar-free option, it is one of the most important ingredients to add in gluten-free baking. It provides a key textural component by creating light, chewy centres and a crispy crust. However, if too much tapioca is used, it can produce the opposite effect of having a gummy texture.

ORGANIC TEFF FLOUR is made from the world's smallest grain as it comes from grass seed, originating in Africa. Like its counterparts, teff is nutrient-dense, especially high in calcium, protein, fibre and iron. It helps boost immunity and aids in circulation whilst supporting bone health. Teff provides a molasses-like nutty, mild flavour profile and lovely brown colour to baked goods. It is also considered a 'heavy flour' like sorghum and millet and absorbs more liquid, so best to mix it with other lighter gluten-free flours and starches with extra liquid to achieve best textural results.

ORGANIC TIGER NUT FLOUR is not a nut as the name suggests, but rather a root vegetable or tuber that grows in Northern Africa and the Mediterranean, lending itself as a great nut and grain substitute in baked goods. High in fibre, iron, potassium, oleic acid and vitamin E, tiger nuts also contain a good balance of fat, carbohydrates and protein. Tiger nut flour is widely used as an almond meal substitute for a nut-free alternative in baking, as its texture is quite gritty (like that of almonds or desiccated coconut) and has a nutty flavour profile. Perfect in denser baked goods like cookies and brownies.

UNSWEETENED APPLE SAUCE is made simply by cooking your peeled apples until soft and pureeing it. If making your own, freeze ½ cup portions in zip lock bags to use when needed for baking. It is a great substitute for oil and any other fruit puree like banana or pumpkin, as it provides a lovely moist texture and natural sweetness.

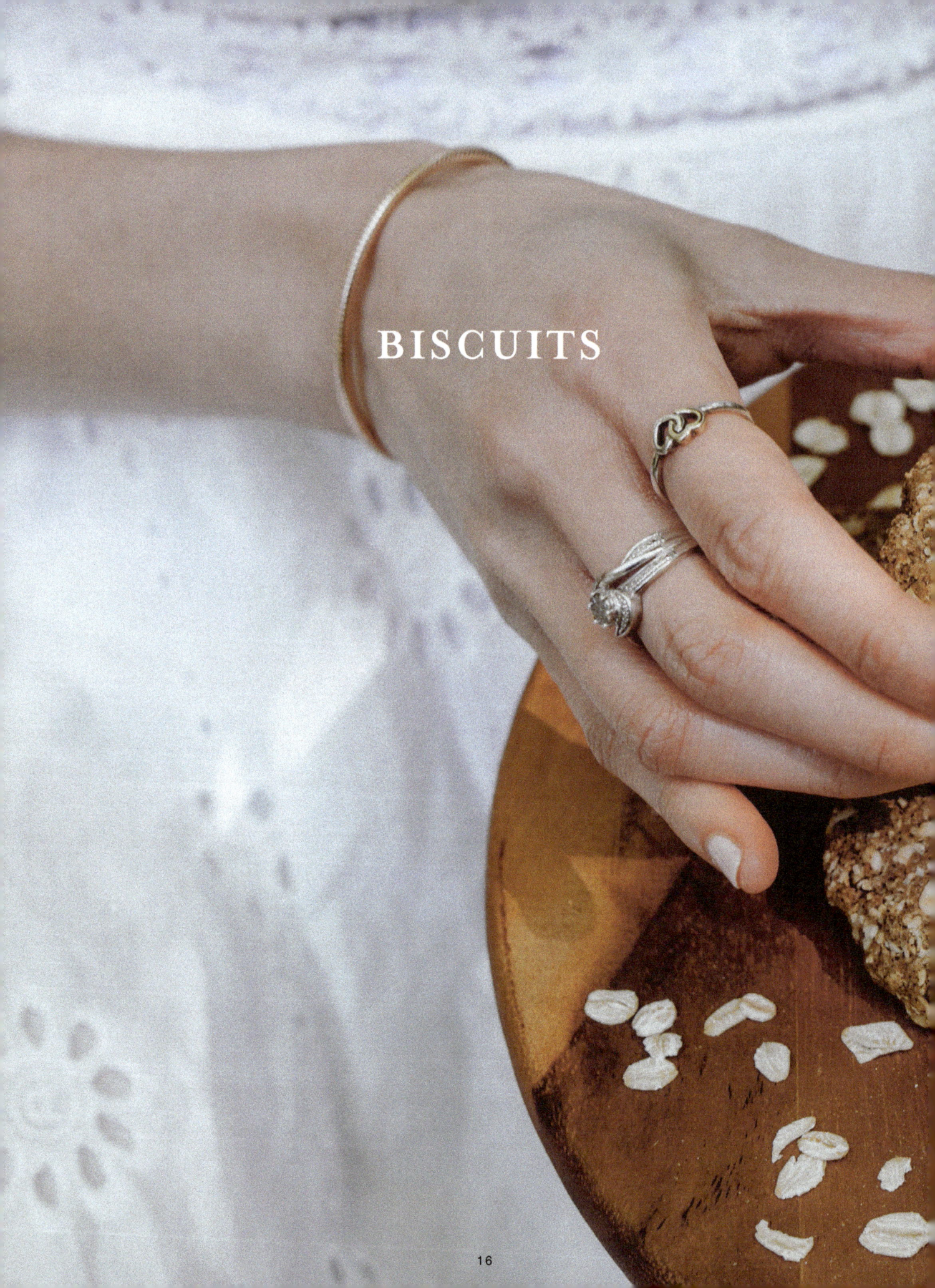
BISCUITS

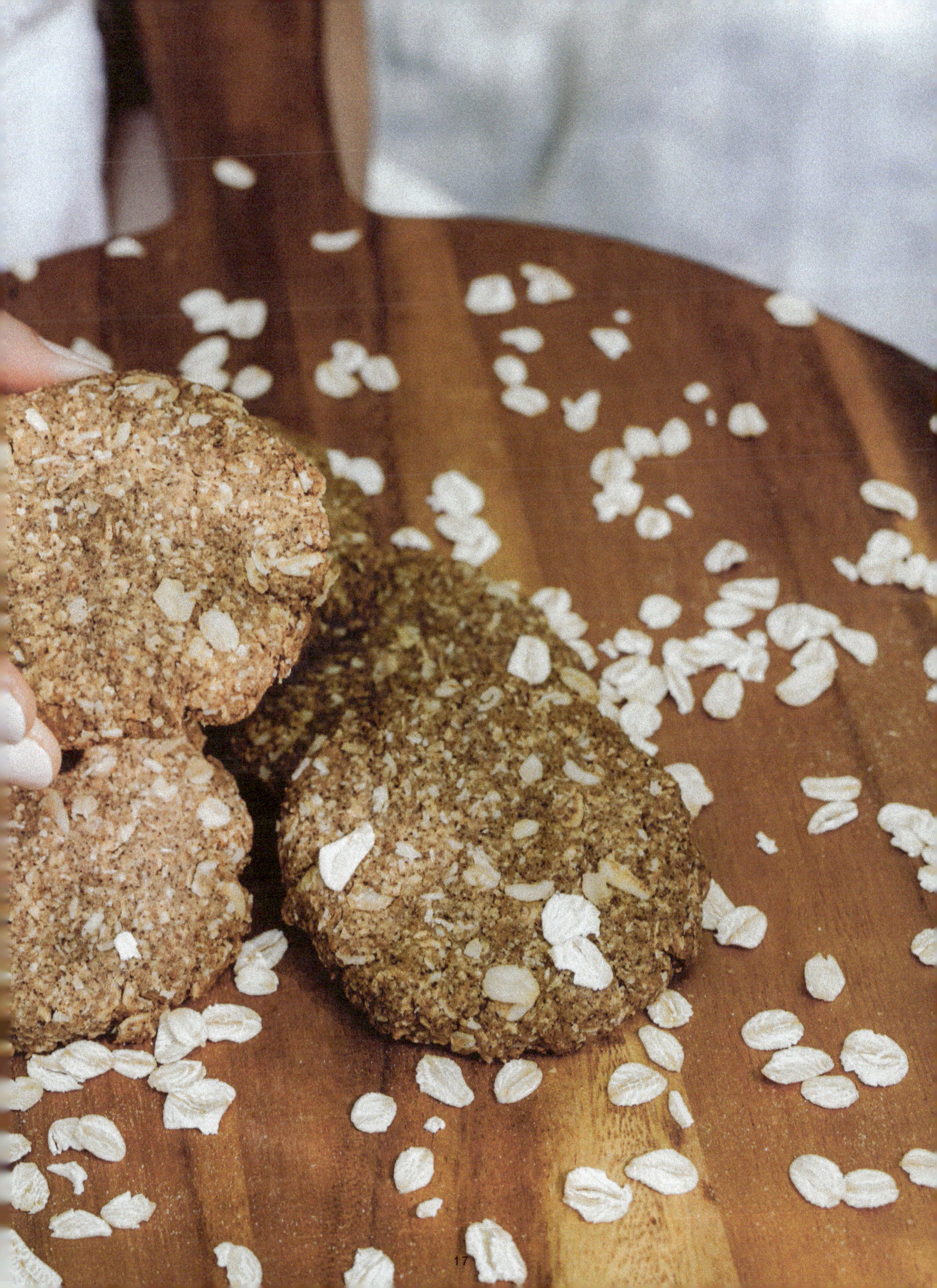

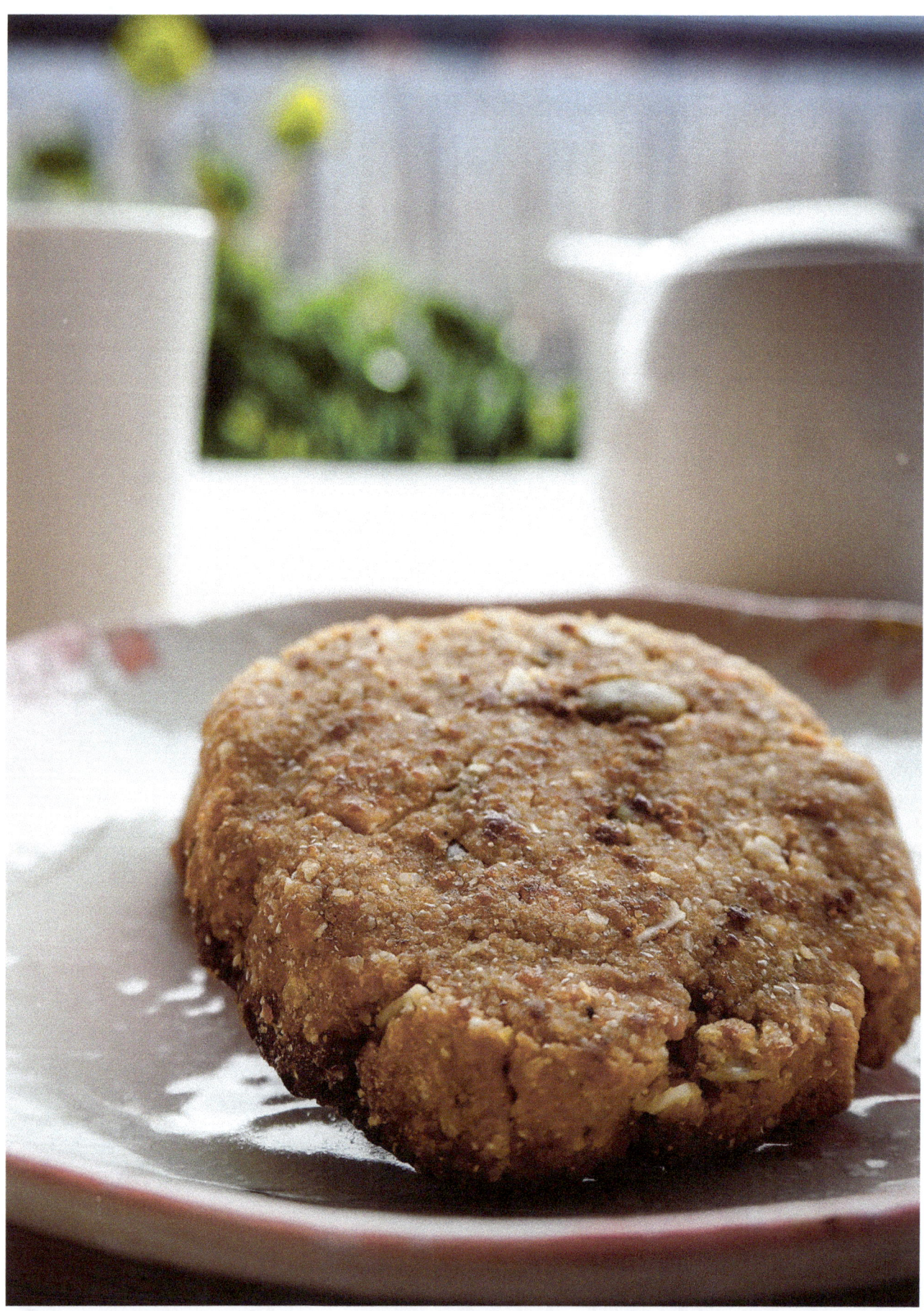

Sweet Potato Biscuits

Makes 12-16 biscuits

These were one of the first types of biscuits I made when I began my alternative baking journey. I have never looked back since, and they are one of my all-time favourite biscuits to make. Eaten warm, they are crispy on the outside but slightly soft and chewy on the inside. The natural sweetness of the sweet potato and the warmth from the ginger are a lovely combination. Satisfy your sweet cravings for morning or afternoon tea with these nutritious gems.

1 cup sweet potato puree
3 tablespoons organic extra virgin coconut oil, solid
¼ cup pure maple syrup
¼ teaspoon salt
¼ teaspoon baking soda
½ teaspoon pure vanilla extract
¼ cup almond flour or tiger nut flour
¼ cup brown rice flour
¼ cup millet flour
2 tablespoons golden flaxseed meal or green banana flour
½ cup oat flour
¼ cup coconut flakes
A handful of pepitas and/or sunflower seeds
1 tablespoon grated fresh ginger (optional)
1 teaspoon coconut sugar for sprinkling on biscuits before baking

Preheat the oven to 163°c and line a baking tray. Peel and rinse a small sweet potato and cut into medium-sized cubes. Cook the sweet potato by either steaming for 10-20 minutes or roasting at 190°c for 30 minutes, turning pieces over at the 15-minute mark. Once cooked, place in a bowl and mash into a puree consistency.

Add organic extra virgin coconut oil, maple syrup, vanilla extract and salt to the hot sweet potato.

Use a stand or electric handheld mixer to beat the sweet potato mixture until creamy. Fold in the flours, baking soda, coconut flakes and pepitas.

Spoon 12-16 balls onto a lined baking tray and flatten them before baking for 35 minutes, turning the tray around at the 15-minute mark.

Remove the tray from the oven and place biscuits on a cooling rack to cool. Once cooled, store them in an airtight container.

RECIPE NOTES

These biscuits are best eaten warm. To reheat, simply place in the oven and heat for 5-10 minutes at 150°c. They also freeze well.

Anzac Biscuits

Makes 20-24 biscuits

These Anzac biscuits are a sure favourite in our home, especially if they are extra crispy for dunking in your tea! Full of the goodness of oats, coconut and packed with prebiotics and fibre, the caramelisation and crunch are oh-so-satisfying. They make for a great mid-morning or afternoon snack and are handy to have in your bag when you are out and about and need an energy boost.

1 cup rolled oats
½ cup desiccated coconut
1 cup Gluten-Free Flour Blend – Option 2

These flour options work well, too:
¼ cup green banana flour or brown rice flour
¼ cup almond flour or tiger nut flour
¼ cup sorghum flour or millet flour
¼ cup tapioca starch

2 tablespoons hemp flour
2 tablespoons golden flaxseed meal
¼ cup coconut sugar
½ teaspoon baking soda
2 tablespoons hot water
100g vegan butter or ⅓ cup organic extra virgin coconut oil or olive oil
¼ cup pure maple syrup
1 teaspoon pure vanilla extract
¼ teaspoon salt
¼ teaspoon cinnamon powder

Preheat the oven to 160°c and line two baking trays. In a mixing bowl, add in the rolled oats, desiccated coconut, flours, flaxseed meal and coconut sugar and stir until combined.

In a small saucepan, melt the vegan butter or add in the oil over medium heat, together with the maple syrup and vanilla extract and whisk until combined. Once the liquid mixture begins to bubble, dissolve the baking soda in 2 tablespoons of hot water and add to the liquid mixture, whisking until it starts to foam and rise.

Immediately pour the hot liquid into the mixing bowl containing the dry ingredients and stir gently until mixed well. The biscuit dough should be quite firm and stiff.

Roll the dough into tablespoon-sized balls and place them on the baking trays, about 2 cm apart. Flatten the balls to about 5 mm thick.

Bake at 160°c for 30 minutes if you prefer them crispy or 180°c for 12-13 minutes if you like them soft and chewy.

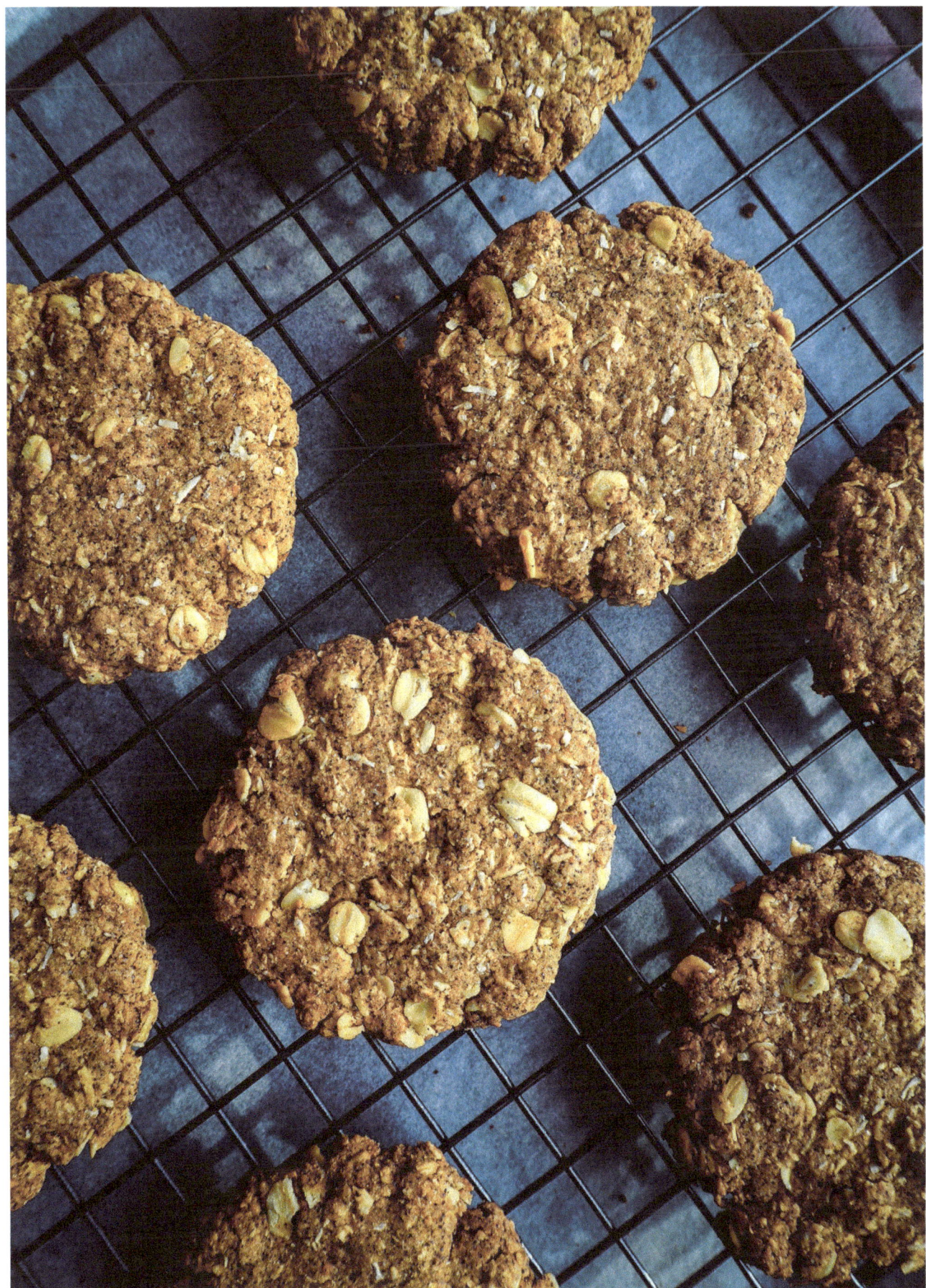

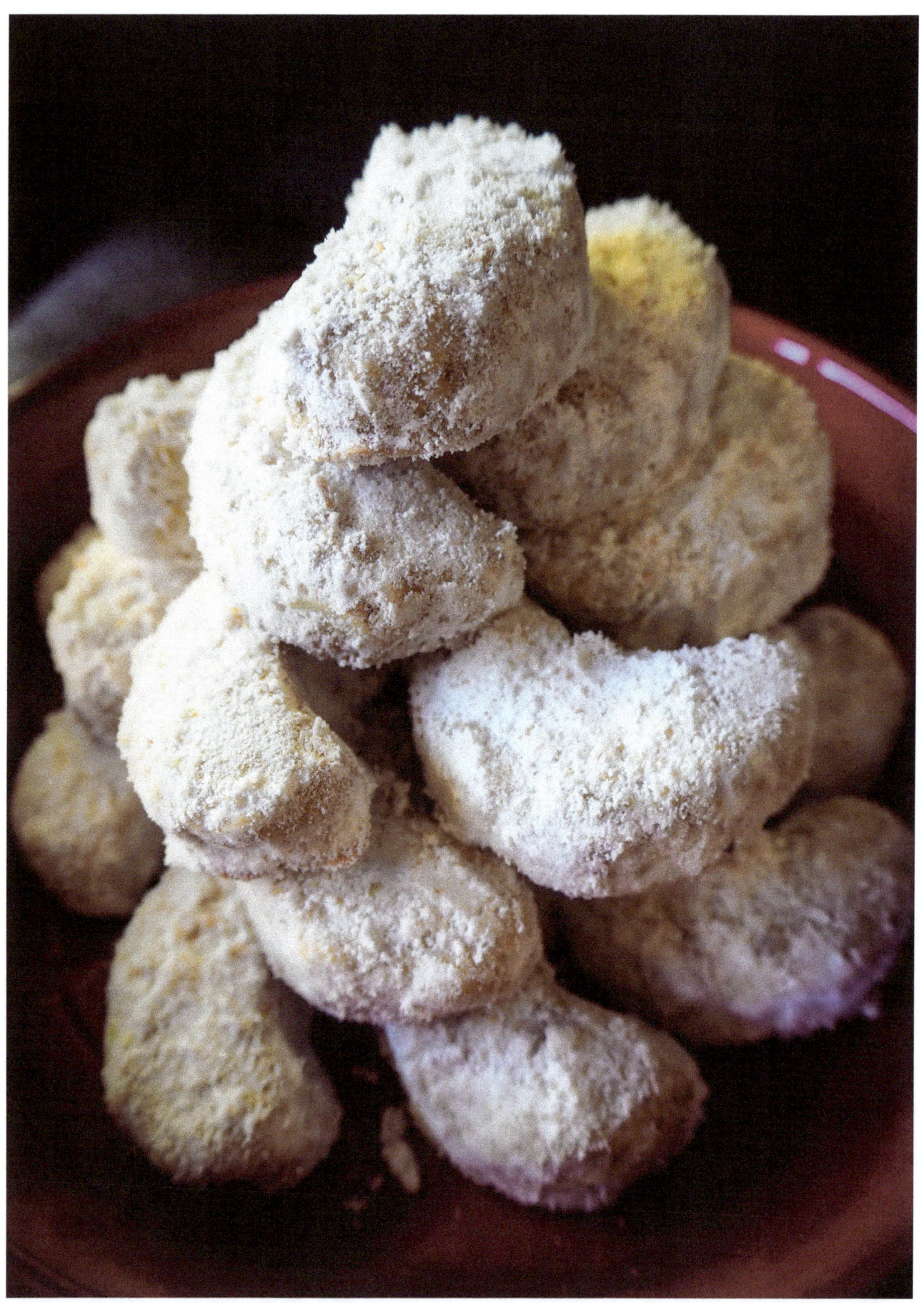

Almond Crescents

Makes 28 biscuits

Almond crescents are reminiscent of Christmas to me, but you will want to bake these beauties at any time of the year. With a soft and slightly chewy texture, the sweet almond flavour is most definitely the star of the show. The simple icing luxuriously coats each crescent, creating a beautifully rich and satisfying biscuit for any occasion.

¾ cup brown rice flour
½ cup sorghum flour or millet flour
1 cup almond flour
¼ cup tapioca starch
2 tablespoons almond butter
2 tablespoons unsweetened almond milk
¼ cup pure maple syrup
2 teaspoons pure vanilla extract
¼ cup organic extra virgin coconut oil, solid
1 teaspoon pure almond extract
¼ teaspoon salt
½ cup blanched almond flakes
The rind of 1 lemon
1 tablespoon lemon juice

ICING (MIXED TOGETHER)
½ cup dairy-free coconut milk powder
1 tablespoon maple sugar (finely ground until icing sugar consistency)

Preheat the oven to 180°c and line a baking tray with baking paper. Process all ingredients (except for the almond flakes) in a food processor until a sticky ball dough is formed. Transfer the dough into a bowl and add in the almond flakes. Knead the dough until the flakes are evenly spread throughout.

Roll the dough into 1 tablespoon-sized balls, then flatten slightly and shape each into crescents. Place them onto the lined baking tray about 2cm apart.

Bake for 15-20 minutes, turning the baking tray around halfway through. Cool completely on a wire rack.

In a small bowl, mix together the coconut milk powder and maple sugar until well combined. Gently toss the crescents in the icing mixture and store in an air-tight container.

RECIPE NOTES

These crescents will be soft and chewy if baking for just 15 minutes. If you prefer a biscuit with more crunch, turn the oven temperature down to 160°c and bake for a further 15 minutes.

Macadamia Cranberry Biscuits

Makes 15 biscuits

Macadamias and cranberries are a sublime combination in a biscuit. The crunch of the macadamias and the subtle tartness and sweetness of the dried cranberries are wonderfully complemented by the maple coconut lemon butter glaze drizzled on top. Deliciously crumbly and moreish, you won't be able to stop at one.

⅓ cup organic extra virgin coconut oil, melted
⅓ cup maple sugar or coconut sugar (mix them both if desired)
1 teaspoon pure vanilla extract
1 free-range egg
¼ cup millet flour or sorghum flour
¼ cup Gluten-Free Flour Blend — Option 1
¼ cupy almond flour or toasted quinoa flour
¼ cup teff flour or chestnut flour
Just under ½ cup oat flour
2 tablespoons golden flaxseed meal
¼ teaspoon baking soda
¼ teaspoon salt
½ cup macadamia nuts, chopped
¼ cup naturally sweetened cranberries

MAPLE COCONUT LEMON BUTTER DRIZZLE (OPTIONAL)
2-3 tablespoons coconut butter
1 teaspoon maple butter or 1 tablespoon pure maple syrup
2 teaspoons lemon juice
1 teaspoon water

Preheat the oven to 180°C. In a mixing bowl, whisk together the coconut oil, maple or coconut sugar, egg and vanilla extract until combined.

Add in the flours, golden flaxseed meal, baking soda and salt. Stir to combine. Fold in the macadamia nuts and cranberries until evenly distributed.

Roll the dough into 15 equal balls and place them on a lined baking tray, flattening them slightly with your fingers. Bake for 16 minutes or until slightly golden brown. Remove from the oven and place them on a cooling rack.

To make the maple coconut lemon butter drizzle, place all ingredients in a bowl and microwave for 10-15 seconds until melted. Alternatively, you can slowly heat the drizzle up in a bowl over a pot of simmering water. Stir thoroughly until drizzle consistency is achieved, adding a bit of water if necessary.

Once biscuits are cool, drizzle the glaze on top. It will set once it is cooled.

RECIPE NOTES

Store biscuits in an airtight container. The biscuits will tend to soften as the glaze adds moisture, so refrigeration is encouraged. However, if you prefer them crispy, reheat them in the oven for 10 minutes at 150°c. Alternatively, you can choose not to have them glazed, which will preserve their crispiness.

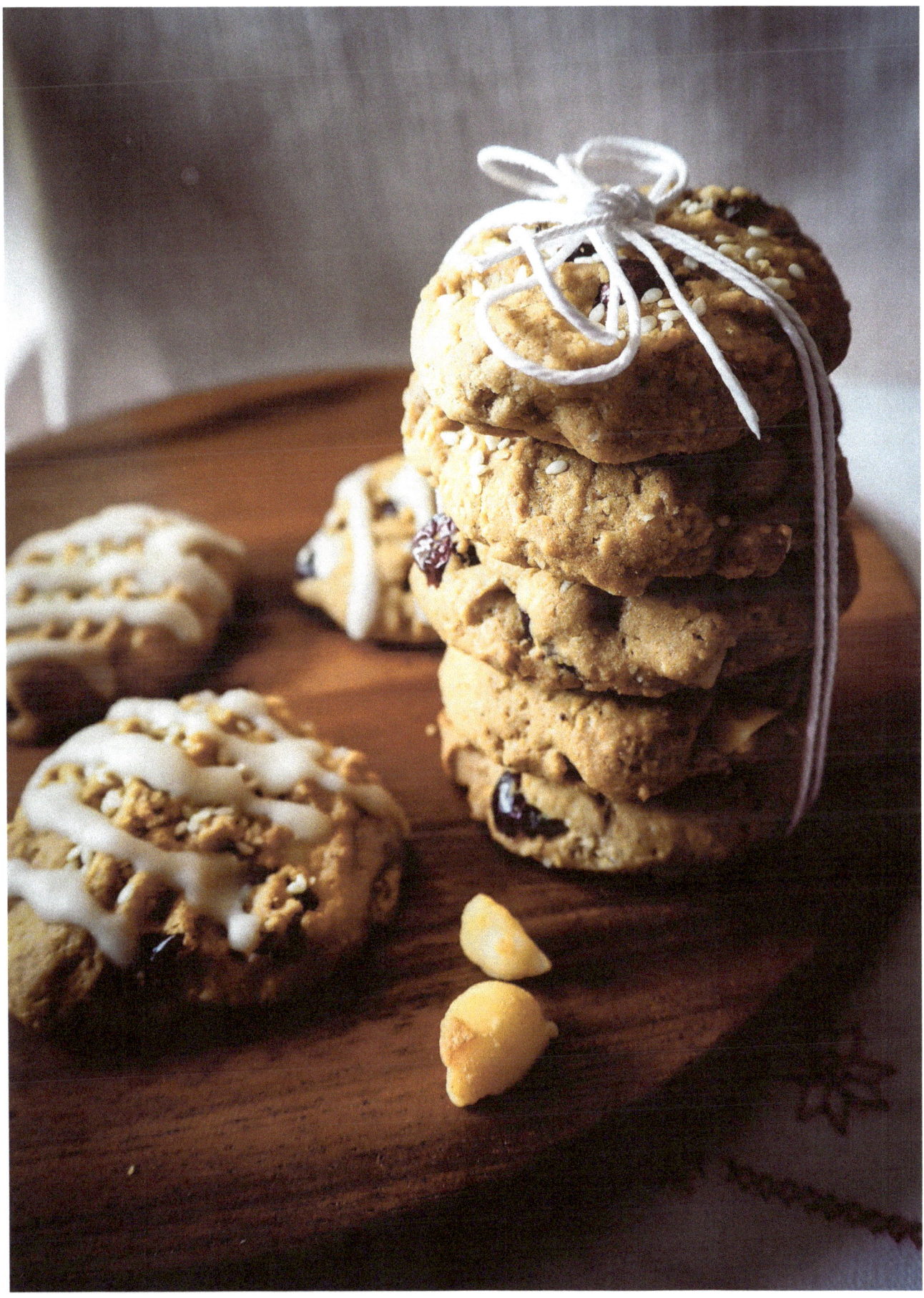

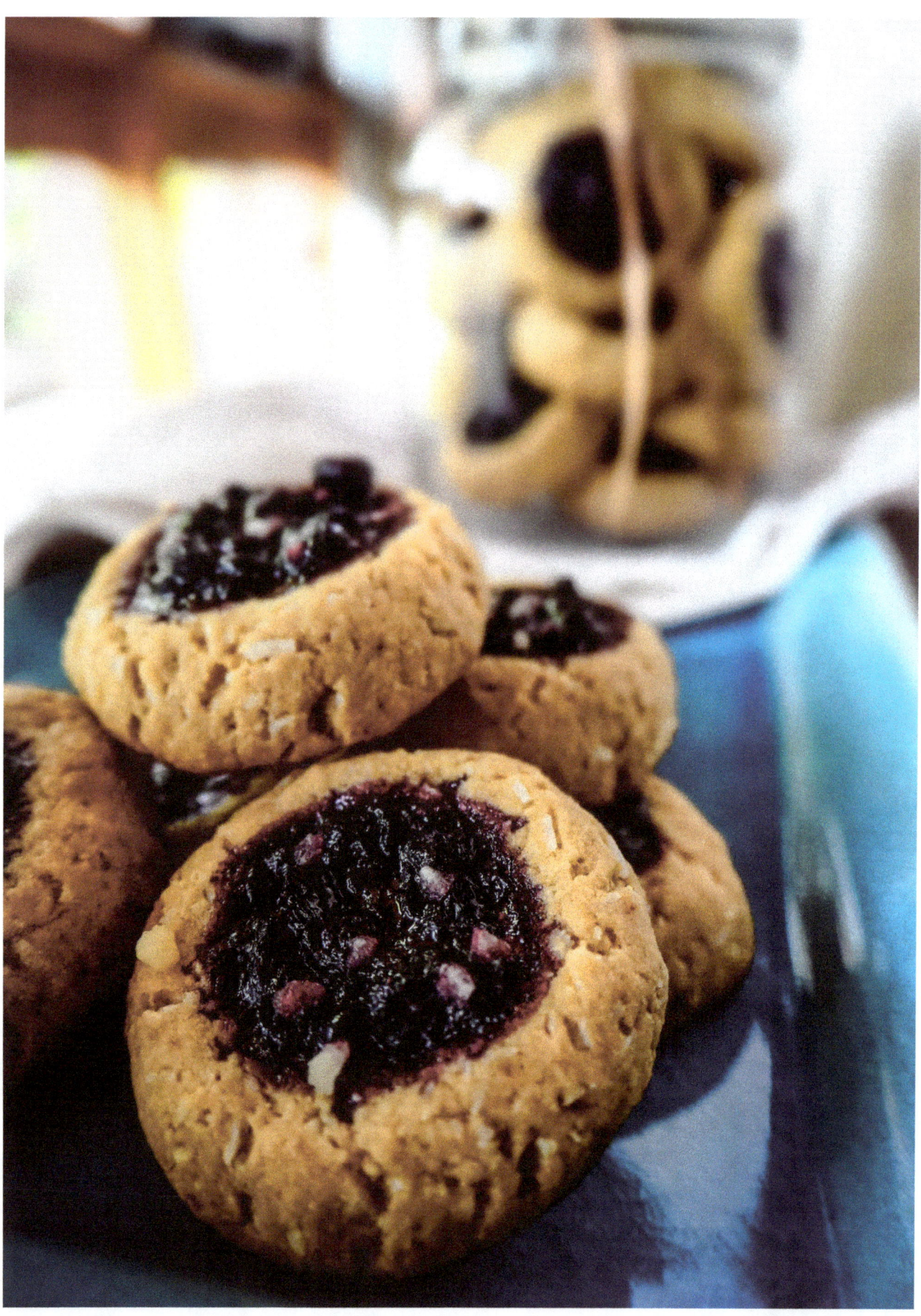

Jam Drop Biscuits

Makes 28 biscuits

These irresistible jam drops feature the flavours of vanilla and coconut, adorned with sweet blueberry jam. Fresh out of the oven, they have just the right combination of crispy edges and soft, gooey centres. Serve them up for an afternoon tea treat with a good cuppa.

⅓ cup organic extra virgin coconut oil, melted
⅓ cup coconut or maple sugar
1 free-range egg
1 ½ teaspoons pure vanilla extract
2 tablespoons pure maple syrup
¾ cup desiccated coconut
½ cup almond flour
¼ cup quinoa flour
¼ cup cassava flour
½ cup Gluten-Free Flour Blend — Option 2
2 tablespoons brown rice flour
¼ teaspoon salt
¼ teaspoon baking soda
Blueberry jam (see recipe on page 103)
Coconut flower nectar sugar to sprinkle on top

Preheat the oven to 175°c. In a mixing bowl, melt the coconut oil and whisk in the coconut sugar, egg, vanilla extract and maple syrup until combined. Add in the desiccated coconut, flours, salt and baking soda, folding through until dough is formed.

Roll tablespoon-sized balls and place on a lined baking tray, about 1 cm apart. Using your thumb or index finger, press into the centre of each ball to create an indent. This will flatten the dough slightly.

Fill each indent with the blueberry jam, then lightly sprinkle some coconut flower nectar sugar on top of each biscuit. Bake in the oven for 20 minutes, turning the tray around half way.

Once out of the oven, transfer the biscuits to a cooling rack to cool down completely. Store the biscuits in an airtight container to maintain freshness.

Gingernut Biscuits

Makes 18-20 biscuits

Ginger is a worthy and very versatile ingredient to always have in your kitchen as it boasts anti-inflammatory and antibacterial properties, just to name a few. These timelessly lovable cookies have a depth of flavour from the warmth of the fresh ginger and the nutty, earthy accents of the chestnut flour. Whether you like them soft and chewy or prefer a crispier texture, these gingernut biscuits are an any-time side-kick to your cuppa.

⅓ cup organic extra virgin coconut oil, melted
1 free-range egg
⅓ cup coconut or maple sugar
1 teaspoon pure vanilla extract
½ teaspoon baking soda
¼ teaspoon cinnamon powder
¼ teaspoon salt
1 teaspoon ginger powder
1 tablespoon freshly grated ginger
3 tablespoons pure maple syrup
½ cup chestnut flour
¼ cup teff flour
¼ cup green banana flour
¼ cup tapioca starch
¼ cup oat flour
¼ cup brown rice flour
¼ cup chopped macadamia nuts
Maple sugar or coconut flower nectar sugar – to sprinkle on top

Preheat the oven to 190°C. In a mixing bowl, whisk together the coconut oil, maple or coconut sugar, egg, vanilla extract and maple syrup until combined. Add in the flours, baking soda, cinnamon, ginger powder, grated ginger and salt. Stir to combine. Fold in the macadamia nuts until they are evenly distributed.

Roll the dough into 18-20 equal balls and place them on a lined baking tray, flattening them slightly. Sprinkle some maple sugar or coconut flower nectar sugar on top of each biscuit.

Bake for 12 minutes or until slightly golden brown. Remove the tray and place the biscuits on a cooling rack, then store them in an airtight container.

RECIPE NOTES

If you prefer the cookies to be crispier, bake at 160°C for 30 minutes instead.

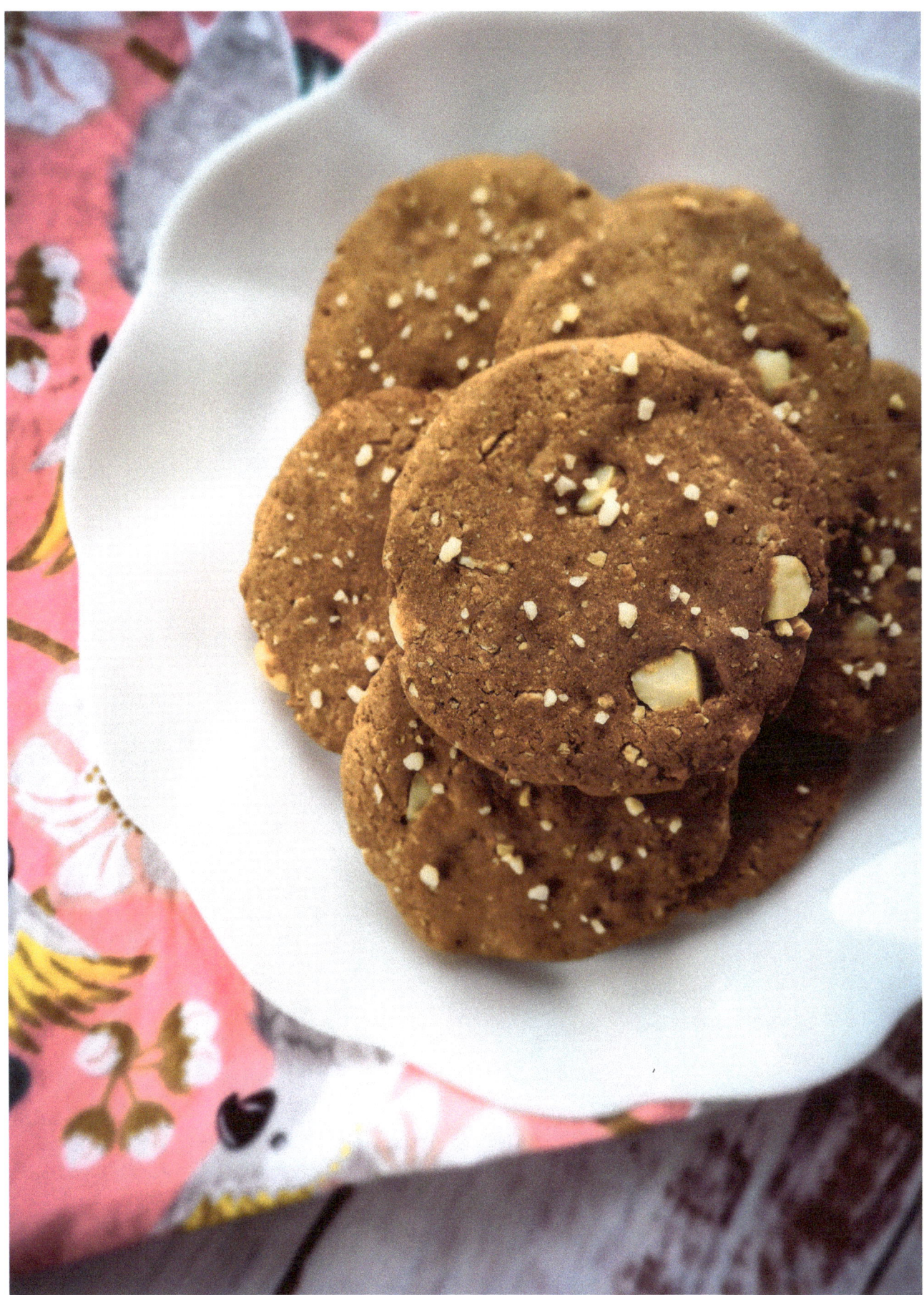

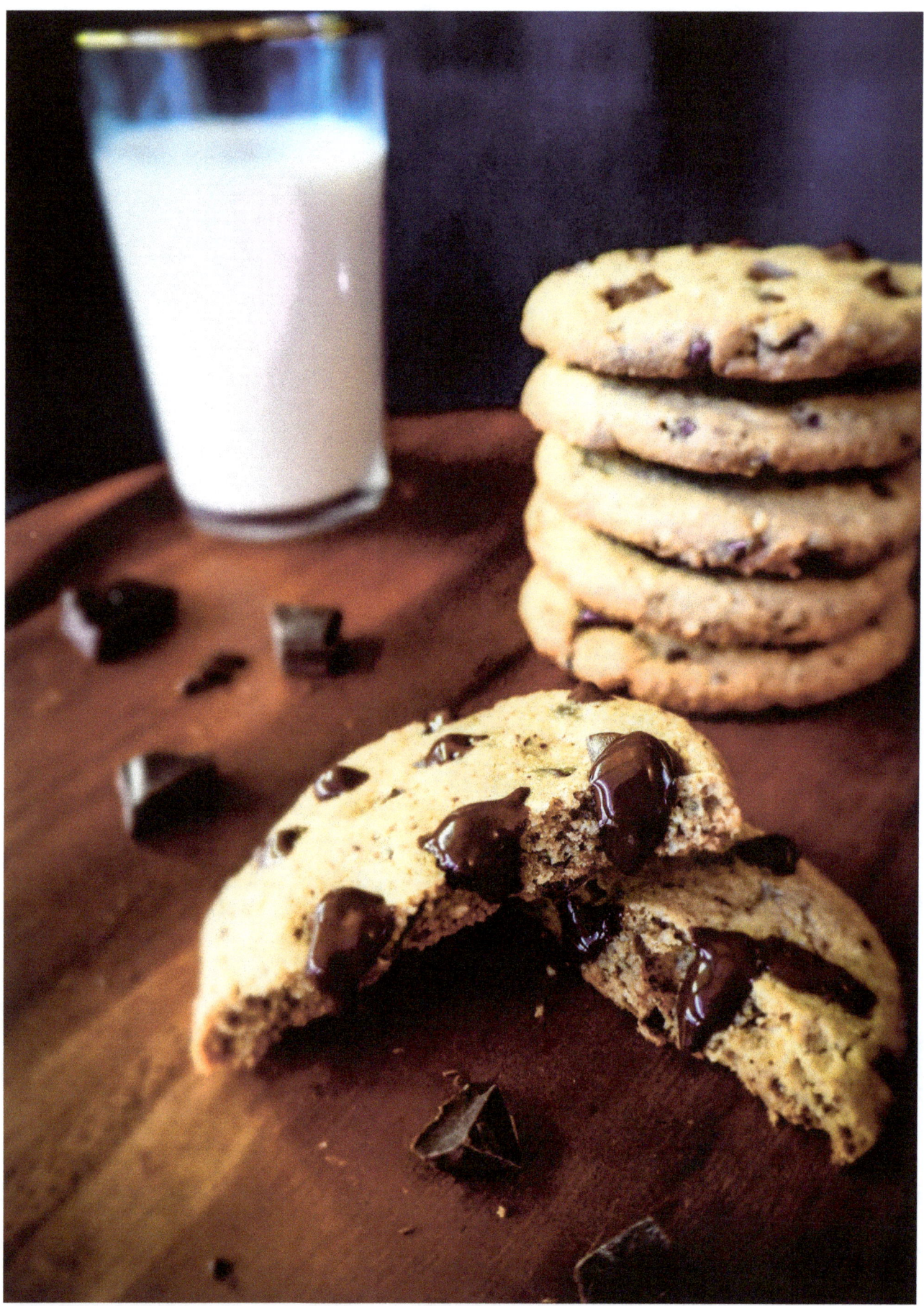

Chocolate Chip Biscuits

Makes 18-20 biscuits

Chocolate chip biscuits are a classic favourite of many. Some prefer them crispy and crumbly, while others prefer them crispy on the outside but soft on the inside. It has taken me a long time to get this right, and boy, have there been countless tastings (not that anyone is complaining), but here they are. My chocolate chip biscuits cross both worlds. Straight out of the oven, they are hot, with crispy edges surrounding a soft centre, dotted with molten chocolate. Once they cool down, they are beautifully crumbly. You get to decide how you want to devour them.

- 1 cup Gluten-Free Flour Blend — Option 2
- ¼ cup almond flour or toasted quinoa flour
- ¼ cup oat flour
- 1 tablespoon coconut flour
- ¼ teaspoon salt
- ¼ teaspoon baking soda
- ¼ cup pure maple syrup
- 2 tablespoons coconut sugar
- 1 free-range egg
- ¼ cup almond butter or sunflower seed butter
- ¼ cup organic extra virgin coconut oil, softened but not melted
- 1 teaspoon pure vanilla extract
- ½ - ¾ cup dark chocolate chips or 90 g 70% dark chocolate block, chopped

Preheat the oven to 180°C. In a mixing bowl, whisk together the coconut oil, maple syrup, coconut sugar, egg, vanilla extract and almond butter until combined. Add in the flour, baking soda and salt. Stir to combine. Fold in the chocolate chips until evenly distributed.

Spoon tablespoon and a half-sized pieces of the dough, roll and place them on a lined tray and flatten them slightly.

Bake for 15-20 minutes or until slightly golden brown. Remove and place on a cooling rack, then store biscuits in an airtight container.

RECIPE NOTES

The longer you bake these biscuits, the crispier and crumblier they will be. If you prefer them crispy on the outside but soft on the inside, bake them for a shorter time.

If you want to replicate how they are straight from the oven, reheat them for 5 minutes at 150°c the next time you eat them. They will become soft on the inside and crispy on the outside.

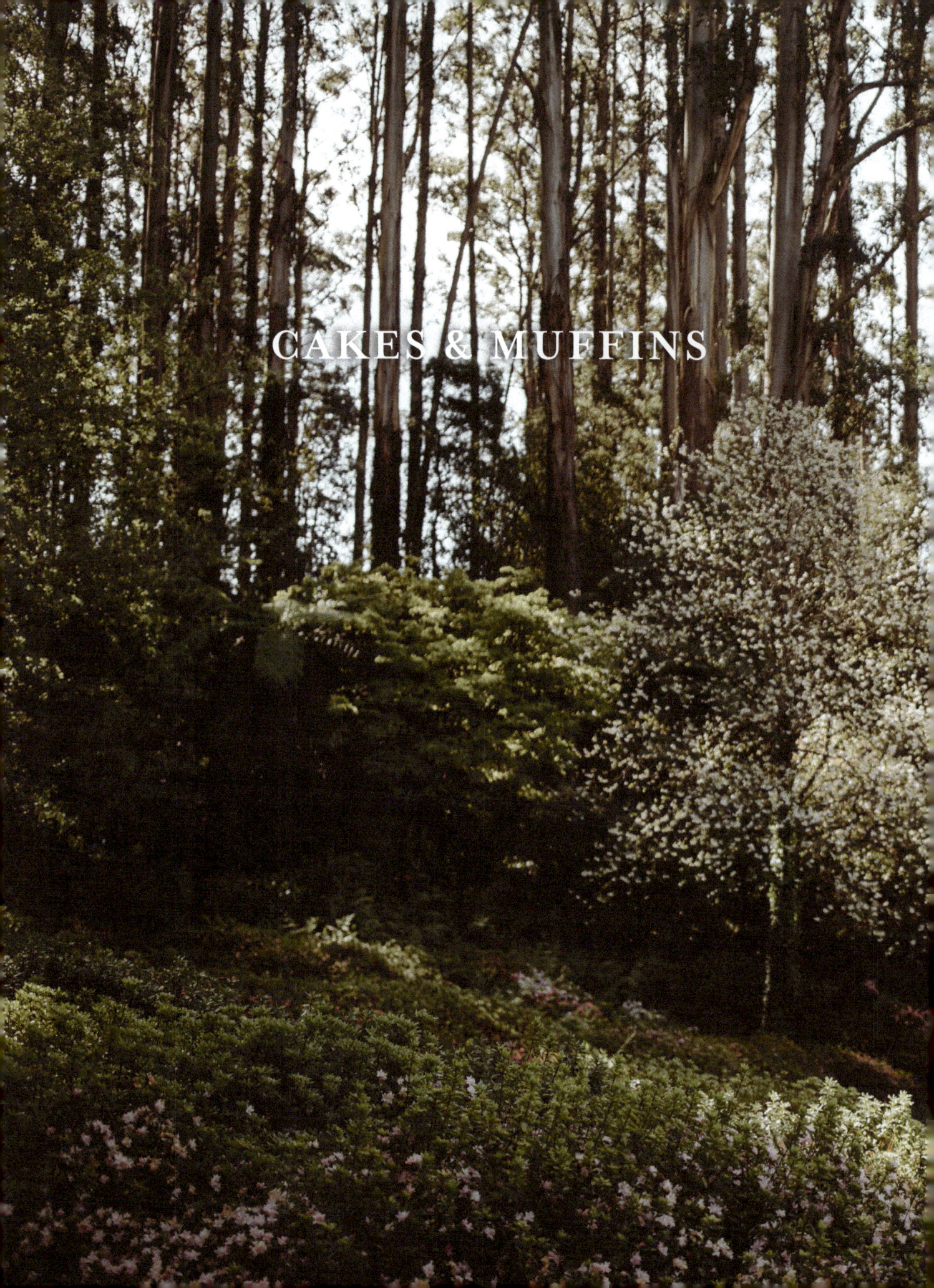
CAKES & MUFFINS

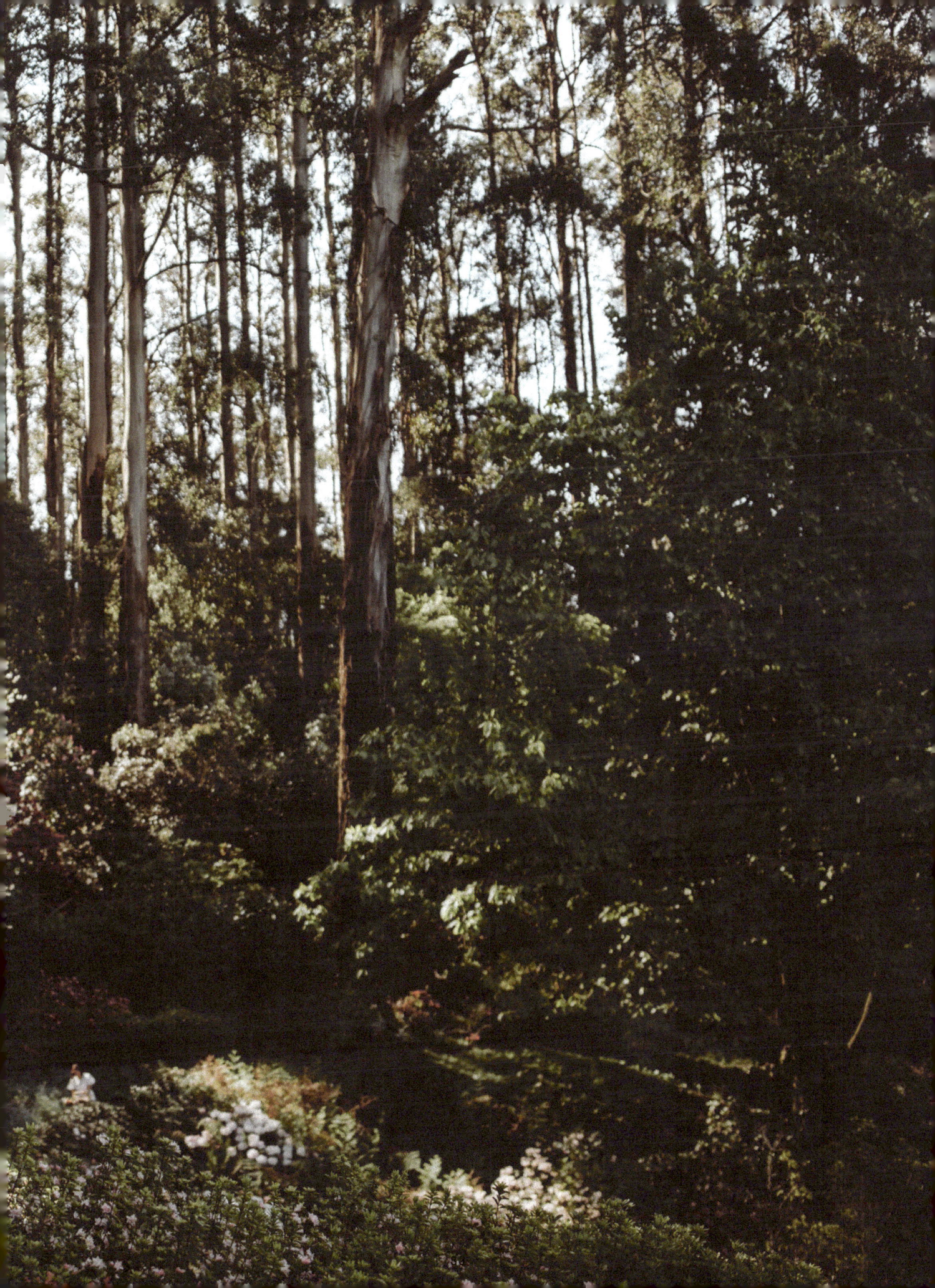

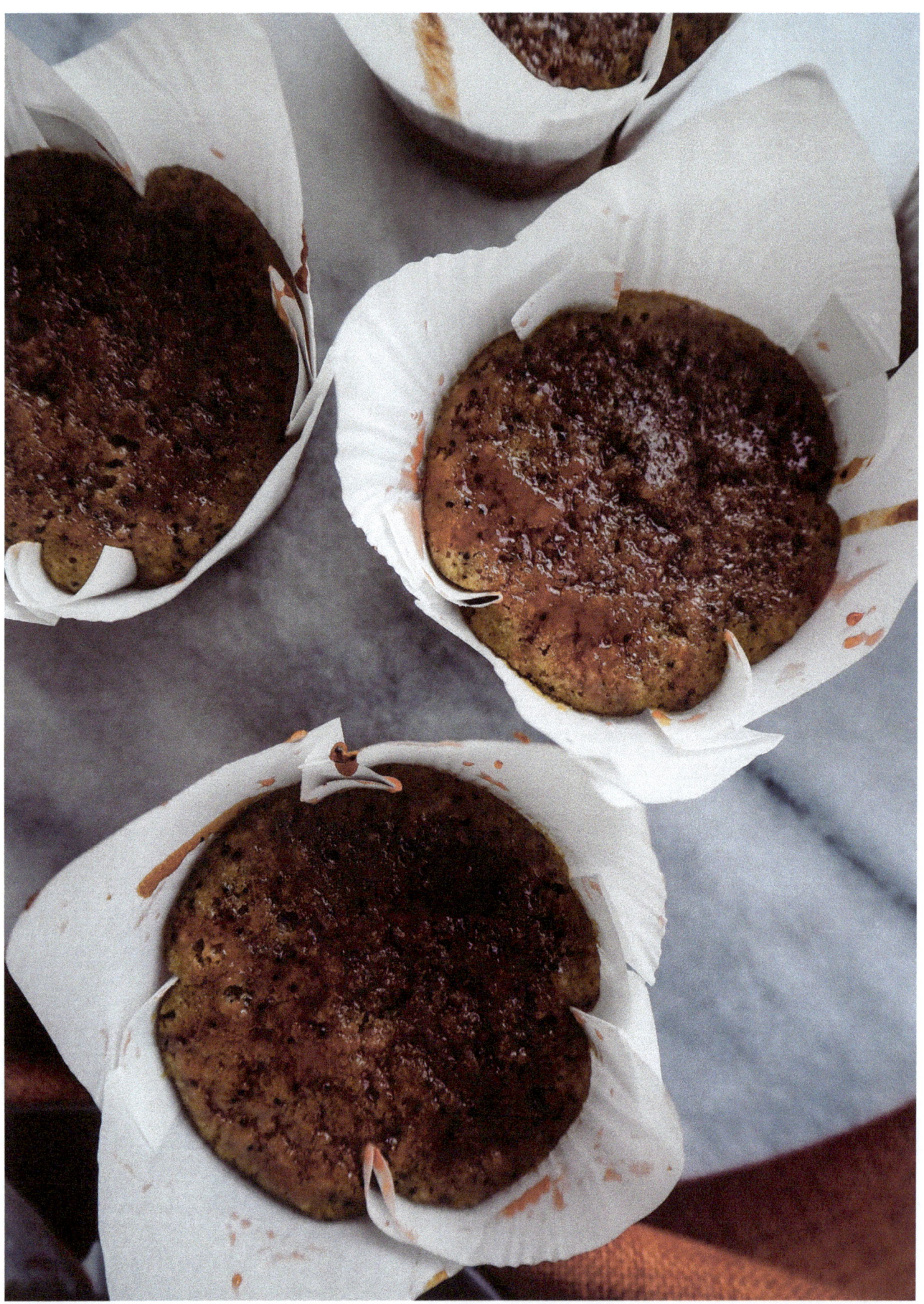

Blood Orange Poppy Seed Muffins

Makes 12 muffins

After a vitamin C pick-me-up? These muffins are light, fresh, zingy and moist with just the right sweetness, paired perfectly with a hot cup of tea. Blood oranges are less acidic than navel oranges and more nutritious with its high level of antioxidants due to its red pigmentation. It also lends a slight raspberry flavour to the muffins, which is just dreamy.

⅓ cup organic extra virgin coconut oil, melted
¼ cup pure maple syrup
2 tablespoons coconut sugar
2 free-range eggs
1 teaspoon pure vanilla extract
4 blood oranges - ¾ cup blood orange juice plus rind of 2 blood oranges
½ cup unsweetened almond milk
½ cup oat flour
¼ cup brown rice flour
¼ cup glutinous rice flour
¼ cup almond flour
¼ cup tiger nut flour or toasted quinoa flour
¼ cup tapioca starch
½ cup sorghum flour
1 teaspoon baking powder
½ teaspoon baking soda
¼ teaspoon salt
1 tablespoon poppy seeds

BLOOD ORANGE SYRUP
Juice from remaining orange
1 tablespoon pure maple syrup

Preheat the oven to 180°c and line a standard 12x muffin mould tin.

Melt coconut oil and whisk in maple syrup, coconut sugar, eggs, vanilla and orange rind together until combined. Add in orange juice and almond milk and mix well.

Add in baking powder, baking soda, salt, poppy seeds and gluten-free flours. Stir to combine well.

Spoon the batter into the lined muffin tin. Bake for 25 minutes or until a skewer inserted comes out clean.

While muffins are in the oven, prepare the orange syrup. Heat up remaining juice from leftover blood oranges with 1 tablespoon of maple syrup and boil until reduced to a syrup consistency. Once muffins are cooling on a wire rack, brush orange syrup on each muffin and serve.

RECIPE NOTES

Feel free to use navel oranges instead of blood oranges.

Muffins freeze well - to reheat, microwave for 50 seconds to warm up.

Breakfast Muffins to Boost

Makes 12 muffins

This is the ideal muffin to have for breakfast, on-the-go, or to add to your kids' lunchboxes. With plenty of hidden fruit and vegetables, it is tasty yet nutritious, giving you and your family the fuel you need to start the day or as a pick-me-up afternoon snack. What's not to love?

½ cup oat flour or millet flour
½ cup almond flour or tiger nut flour or toasted quinoa flour
½ cup brown rice flour or sorghum flour
¼ cup green banana flour or teff flour
¼ cup tapioca starch
1 teaspoon baking powder
1 teaspoon baking soda
½ teaspoon apple cider vinegar
¼ teaspoon salt
½ teaspoon cinnamon
1 cup pumpkin puree or sweet potato puree or 2 mashed bananas
2 free-range eggs
¼ cup organic extra virgin coconut oil, melted
¼ cup almond butter
¼ cup pure maple syrup
1 teaspoon pure vanilla extract
1 carrot, shredded
1 apple, shredded (add a squeeze of lemon juice to stop browning)
1 zucchini, shredded (juice squeezed out)
¼ cup pecans (to top)
¼ cup shredded or flaked coconut
¼ cup dried sultanas/cranberries/blueberries (optional)

Preheat the oven to 180°C and line a 12-hole muffin tin.

Whisk the puree of choice, eggs, coconut oil, almond butter, maple syrup, vanilla extract and apple cider vinegar together until combined.

Add in the flours, baking powder, baking soda, salt and cinnamon and stir to mix through.

Add in the shredded carrot, apple, zucchini and dried fruit and stir to combine.

Spoon the batter into the lined muffin tin. Top each muffin with pecans and shredded or flaked coconut. Bake for 25-35 minutes until a skewer inserted into the centre of a muffin comes out clean.

Once the muffins are cooked, remove and place on a wire rack to cool.

RECIPE NOTES

These muffins are best eaten warm and served with some butter or vegan butter. They also freeze well. To reheat from frozen, microwave for 50 seconds to 1 minute.

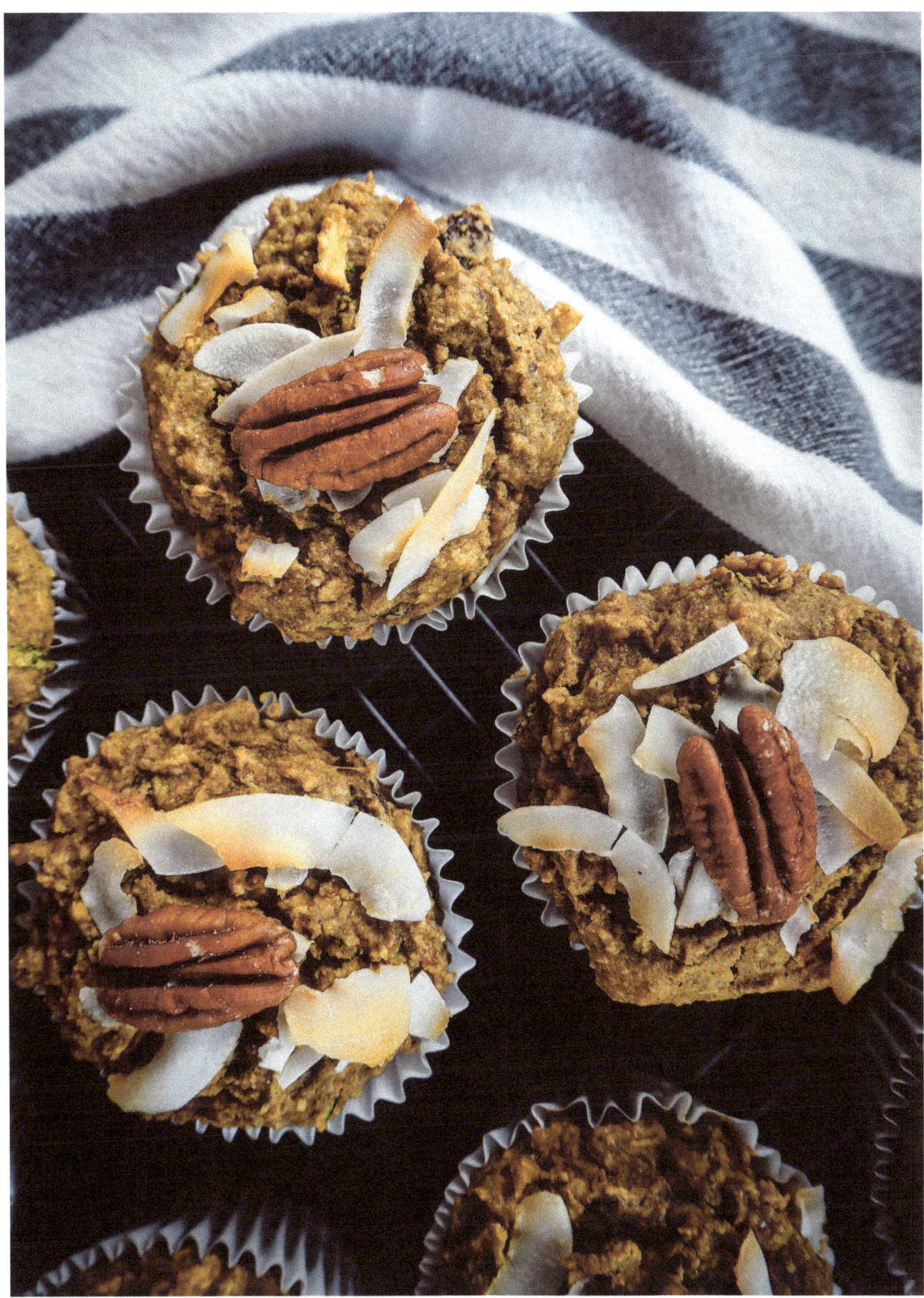

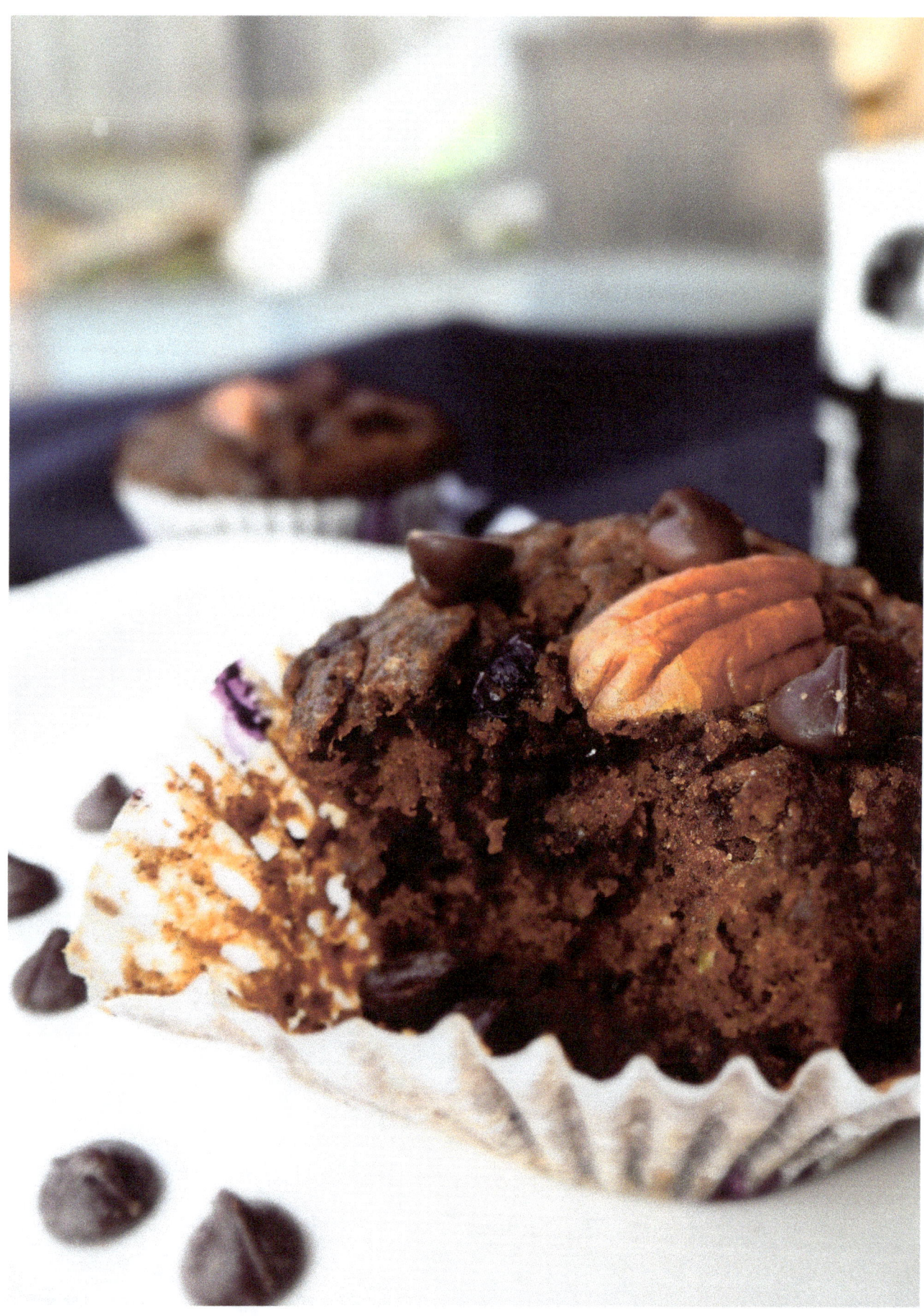

Double Chocolate Banana Zucchini Blueberry Muffins

Makes 12 muffins

These muffins are absolutely delicious as an afternoon snack or dessert. Packed with antioxidants, fibre and nutritional goodness, they sure hit the spot when you are craving something chocolatey and satisfying. The kids won't even know there are vegetables in them!

⅓ cup organic extra virgin coconut oil, melted
¼ cup pure maple syrup
1 free-range egg
1 teaspoon pure vanilla extract
1 cup shredded zucchini, squeezed
3 large ripe bananas or 4 small bananas, mashed
¼ cup almond butter
½ cup unsweetened almond milk
1 teaspoon apple cider vinegar
½ teaspoon cinnamon powder
¼ teaspoon salt
1 teaspoon baking powder
½ teaspoon baking soda
¼ cup cacao powder
½ cup teff flour
½ cup oat flour
¼ cup brown rice flour
¼ cup quinoa flour
¼ cup tapioca starch
2 tablespoons hemp flour
1 cup fresh or frozen blueberries
90 g of 70% dark choc block, chopped into pieces or ½ cup dark chocolate chips

Preheat the oven to 180°c and line a standard 12x muffin mould tin.

Melt coconut oil and whisk in maple syrup, egg and vanilla together until combined. Add in almond butter and almond milk and mix well. Mash bananas and add in, together with shredded zucchini.

Add in cinnamon, baking powder, baking soda, salt, cacao powder, apple cider vinegar and gluten-free flours. Stir to combine well.

Add in blueberries and chopped chocolate or chocolate chips and stir till evenly mixed.

Spoon the batter into the lined muffin tin and top with pecans. Bake at 180°c for 30-40 minutes or until a skewer inserted comes out clean.

RECIPE NOTES

Muffins freeze well - microwave for 50 seconds to 1 minute to warm up.

Lemon Yoghurt Tea Cake

Makes 10 serves

The perfect cake for an afternoon tea with friends and family, this lemon pound cake is moist, lemony and incredibly delicious. As the saying goes, the icing on the cake here is the lemon glaze which just makes you want to reach for another piece of cake, or maybe lick the icing bowl!

3 free-range eggs
⅓ cup pure maple syrup
⅓ cup extra virgin coconut oil, melted
¼ cup coconut sugar
2 teaspoons pure vanilla extract (1 teaspoon if coconut yoghurt is vanilla flavoured)
The rind of 2 small lemons or 1 big lemon
4 tablespoons lemon juice
1 cup unsweetened coconut yoghurt (vanilla flavoured is optional)
1 cup oat flour
¼ cup green banana flour
¼ cup brown rice flour or sorghum flour
¼ cup almond flour/meal
¼ cup tapioca starch or arrowroot starch
2 tablespoons millet flour
1 teaspoon baking powder
½ teaspoon baking soda
¼ teaspoon salt

LEMON GLAZE
¼ cup organic coconut cream or 3-4 tablespoons of coconut butter, melted
2 tablespoons lemon juice
3 tablespoons pure maple syrup
Pinch of salt
½ to 1 teaspoon of water (if needed)

Preheat the oven to 180°C. Grease and line a 13.5 cm x 26.5 cm cake loaf tin.

Melt coconut oil and whisk in maple syrup, coconut sugar, eggs and vanilla until combined. Add in lemon rind, lemon juice and coconut yoghurt and whisk together well.

Add in the gluten-free flours, baking powder, baking soda and salt, and stir together until combined.

Pour cake batter into the loaf tin and bake for 60 minutes to 1 hour 10 minutes or until a skewer inserted into the centre of the cake comes out clean.

Once out of the oven, wait for 10 minutes to cool before removing it onto a cooling rack to cool completely.

While the cake is cooling, make the lemon glaze. If using coconut cream, heat all ingredients in a small saucepan and simmer until thickened and caramelised. If using coconut butter, add all ingredients into a microwavable bowl and heat for 30 seconds. Add a bit of water to create desired consistency for drizzling. Top cake with glaze and toasted almond flakes or desiccated coconut.

Wait until the cake has cooled down completely before cutting and serve.

RECIPE NOTES

This cake freezes well. To reheat, microwave for 50 seconds to warm up.

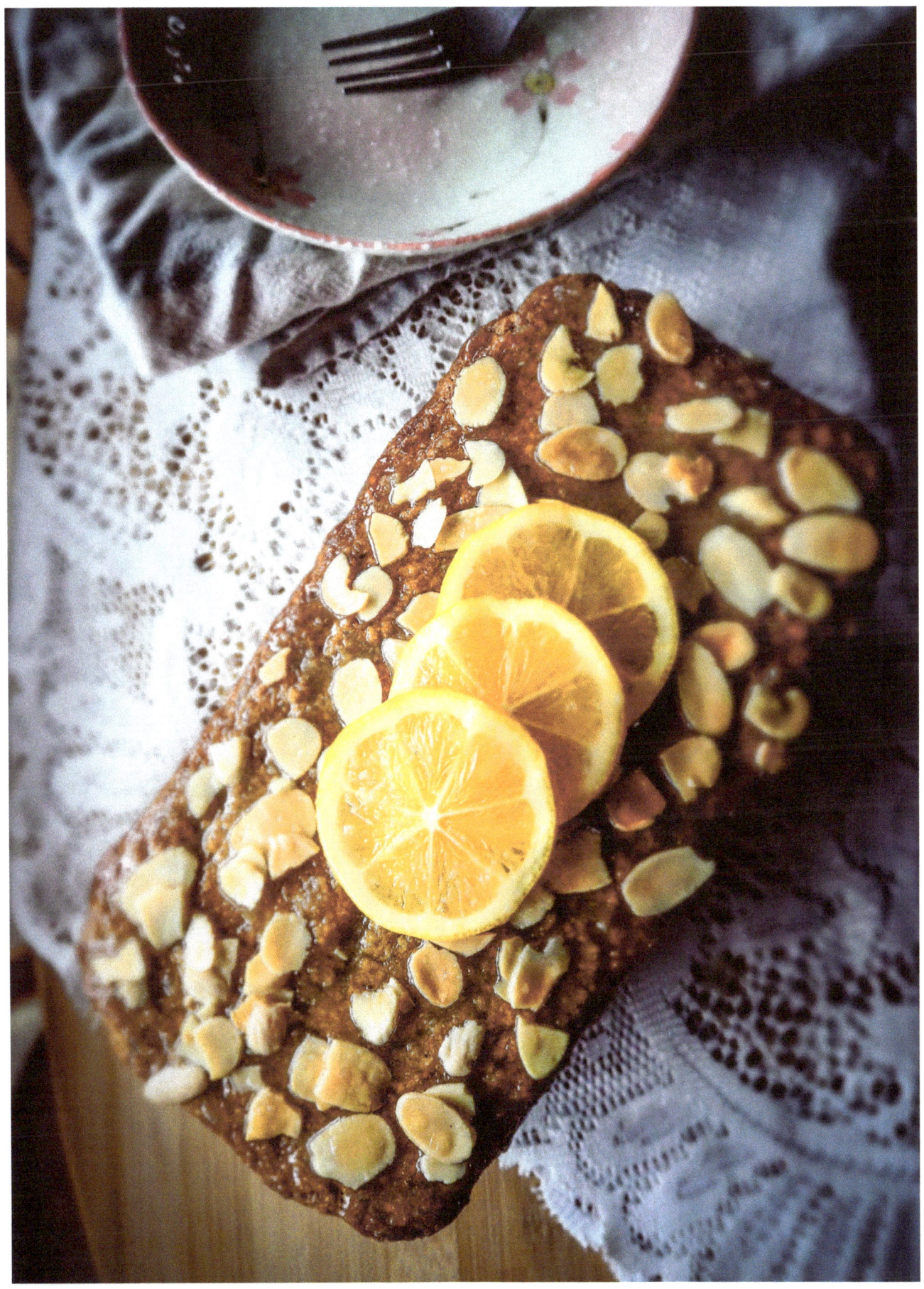

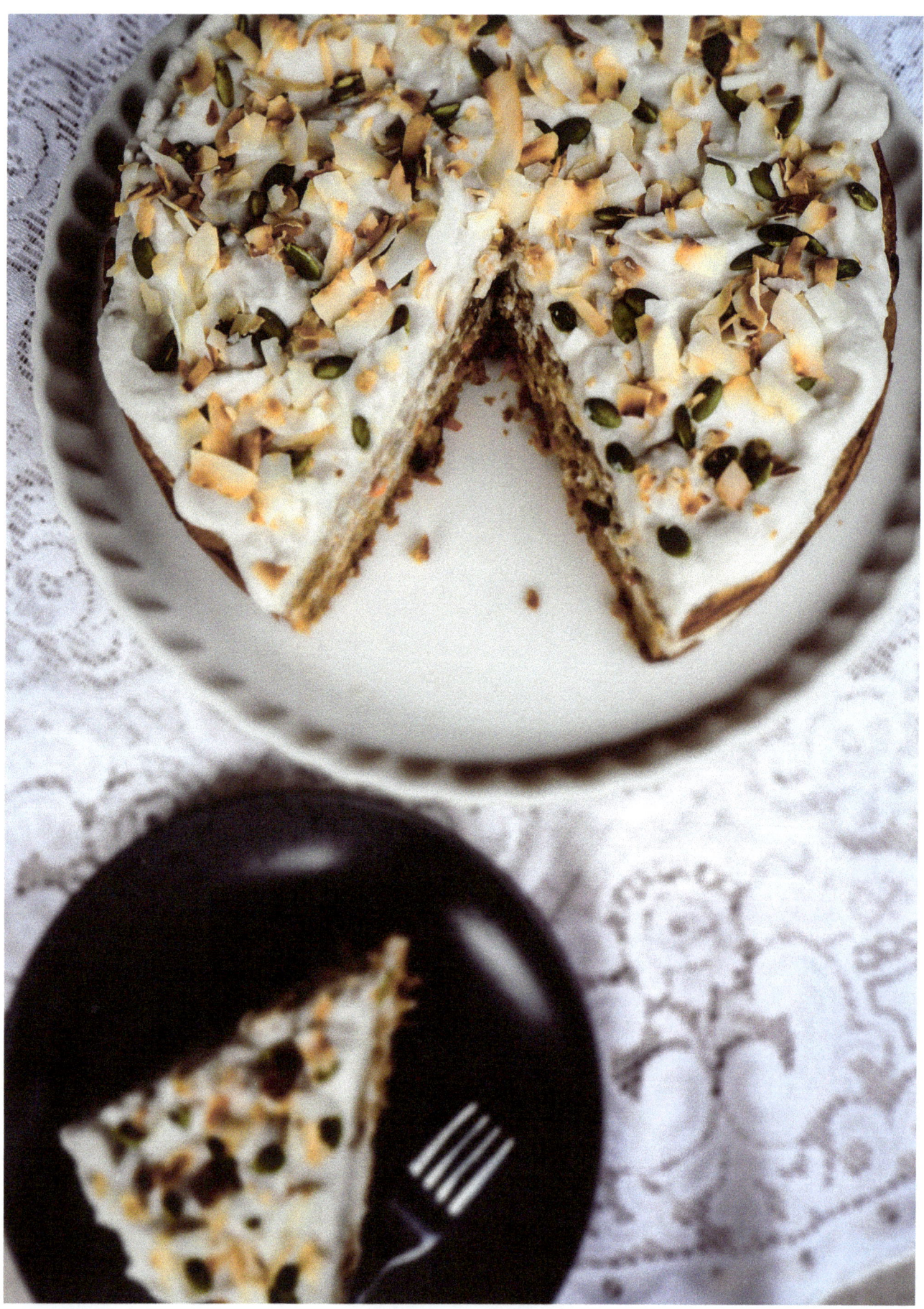

Carrot Cake

Makes 12 serves

Carrot cake has always been one of my favourite cakes to eat. There is something beautiful and comforting about the combination of carrots, spices, pops of sultanas together in a moist cake, layered with a delicious vanilla cream-cheese frosting. With subtle notes of apple, ginger and coconut, and likened to a succulent mud cake in its density, this carrot cake-variation is rich in flavour yet surprisingly refreshing.

⅓ cup olive oil or organic extra virgin coconut oil, melted
¼ cup pure maple syrup
¼ cup coconut sugar
2 free-range eggs
3 large or 4 small carrots, grated but not squeezed
1 cup unsweetened coconut yoghurt (vanilla flavoured)
½ cup heaped unsweetened applesauce
½ cup unsweetened almond milk
1 teaspoon pure vanilla extract
½ teaspoon apple cider vinegar
½ teaspoon cinnamon powder
⅛ teaspoon nutmeg powder
1 tablespoon freshly grated ginger or 1 teaspoon ginger powder
The rind of 1 lemon
2 tablespoons golden flaxseed meal
1 teaspoon baking powder
½ teaspoon baking soda
¼ teaspoon salt
¼ cup dried cranberries or sultanas (sulphite free)
½ cup pecans, chopped
½ cup oat flour
1 ¼ cups Gluten-Free Flour Blend — Option 2
¼ cup chestnut flour or toasted quinoa flour
¼ cup almond flour or tiger nut flour

CREAM CHEESE FROSTING
Refer to Dairy-Free 'Mascarpone' — Option 1 in the Tiramisu Recipe on page 72.

Preheat the oven to 175°c and grease and line the bottom of two 23 cm round cake tins with removable bases.

In a mixing bowl, whisk together the melted coconut oil or olive oil, eggs, maple syrup, coconut sugar and vanilla extract until combined. Stir in the applesauce, almond milk, coconut yoghurt, grated carrots, ginger powder or fresh ginger, apple cider vinegar, cinnamon powder, nutmeg powder and lemon rind until mixed through.

Add in the flaxseed meal, flours, baking powder, baking soda and salt and mix well. Lastly, add in the dried cranberries or sultanas and chopped pecans and stir until evenly distributed.

Transfer the batter evenly across both cake tins and bake for 40-50 minutes, or until a skewer inserted into the centre of the cake comes out clean. Once out of the oven, let it sit in the tin for 10 minutes before transferring to a cooling rack to cool completely.

Once the cake has cooled completely, spread the 'cream cheese frosting' on top of the first layer. Then, place the second cake on top and spread the remaining frosting over the cake. Decorate with pepitas and toasted coconut flakes.

RECIPE NOTES

This cake is best eaten on the day it is made, as freezing it would mean needing to reheat the cake, however, reheating the frosting is not ideal.

Lamingtons with Raspberry Jam

Makes 20 slices

Lamingtons — a classic Australian sweet treat that we have all come to know and love. We have mixed things up a bit here, with the addition of a zesty raspberry jam, sandwiched by moist vanilla cake that is bathed in creamy chocolate and rolled in desiccated coconut. These tasty morsels are bound to hit the spot!

VANILLA CAKE BASE
¼ cup organic extra virgin coconut oil
½ cup organic applesauce
200 ml unsweetened almond milk
Juice of ½ lemon or 1 ½ teaspoons apple cider vinegar
3 large or 4 small free-range eggs, separated
2 teaspoons pure vanilla extract
¼ cup pure maple syrup
4 tablespoons coconut sugar
1 cup almond flour
½ cup sorghum flour or millet flour
1 ¼ cups Gluten-Free Flour Blend – Option 1
1 heaped teaspoon baking powder
½ teaspoon baking soda
¼ teaspoon salt

CHOCOLATE ICING
2 tablespoons pure maple syrup
⅛ cup boiling water
¼ cup cacao powder
2 tablespoons organic extra virgin coconut oil, melted
3 tablespoons unsweetened almond milk
1 tablespoon maple sugar
1 teaspoon pure vanilla extract
Pinch of salt
1 ½ -2 cups unsweetened desiccated coconut to coat

VANILLA CAKE BASE
Preheat the oven to 180°c and line a 19.5 cm x 29.5 cm cake tin. Pour the almond milk in a bowl along with the lemon juice or apple cider vinegar, stir and let the mixture sit for 5 minutes (this acts as buttermilk).

In a separate bowl, whisk together the melted coconut oil, egg yolks, vanilla extract, maple syrup, coconut sugar, applesauce and milk mixture until well combined. Add the flours, baking powder, baking soda and salt and mix well.

In another bowl, beat the egg whites until stiff peaks form. Fold the beaten egg whites into the batter gently until just combined.

Transfer the batter into the cake tin and bake for 25-35 minutes, or until a skewer inserted into the centre of the cake comes out clean. Once out of the oven, let it sit in the tin for 5 minutes before transferring to a cooling rack to cool completely.

CHOCOLATE ICING
In a bowl, mix all of the ingredients together (except for the desiccated coconut) and whisk until smooth. Set aside to cool.

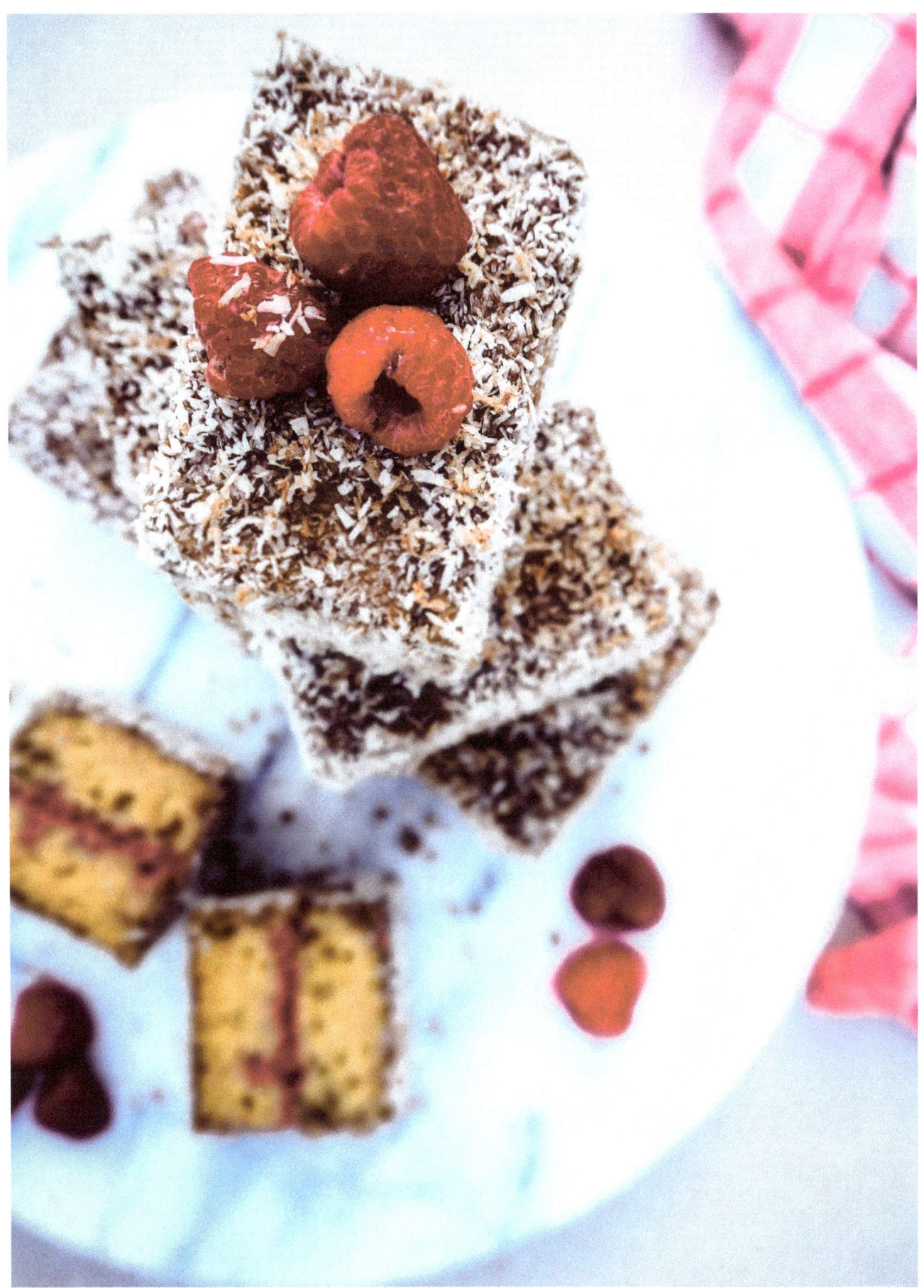

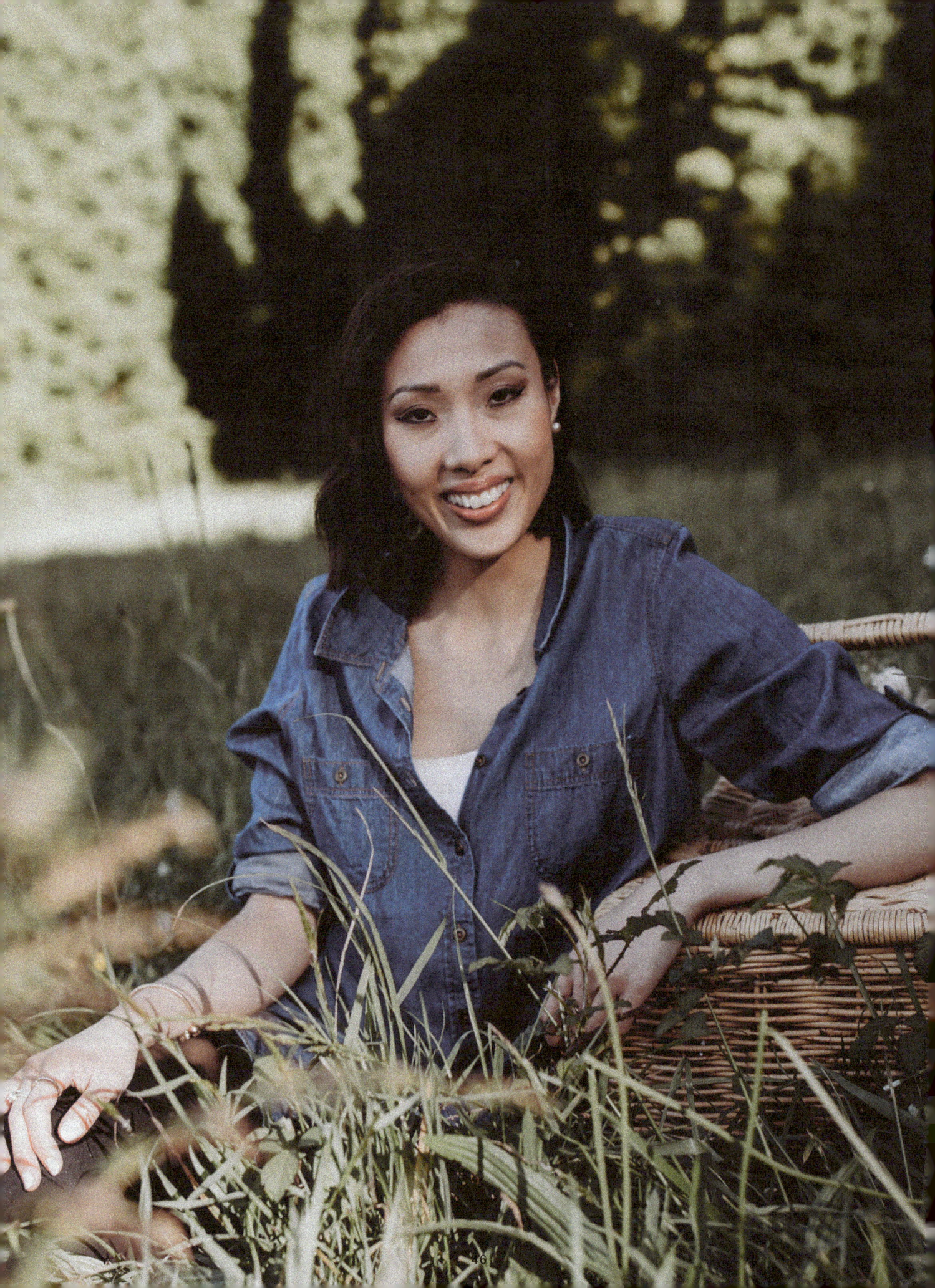

Lamingtons with Raspberry Jam Continued —

RASPBERRY JAM
1 ½ cups fresh or frozen organic raspberries
¼ cup water
½ teaspoon lemon rind
3 tablespoons pure maple syrup
1 tablespoon tapioca starch
½ teaspoon pure vanilla extract
Pinch of salt

RASPBERRY JAM
Add all ingredients to a saucepan and cook on medium heat, stirring frequently until jam thickens. Remove from heat and let it cool completely.

ASSEMBLY
Once the vanilla cake has cooled down completely, cut the cake into 20 equal portions. Cut each portion in half and spread a generous amount of raspberry jam on one side, then sandwich the jam layer with the other cake portion. Repeat this process with all 20 slices.

Dip each side of the lamingtons into the chocolate icing mixture to coat completely, then, roll it in the desiccated coconut. Repeat this process until all the lamingtons are coated in the chocolate icing and desiccated coconut.

Allow them to set for around 10 minutes and then they are ready to be eaten!

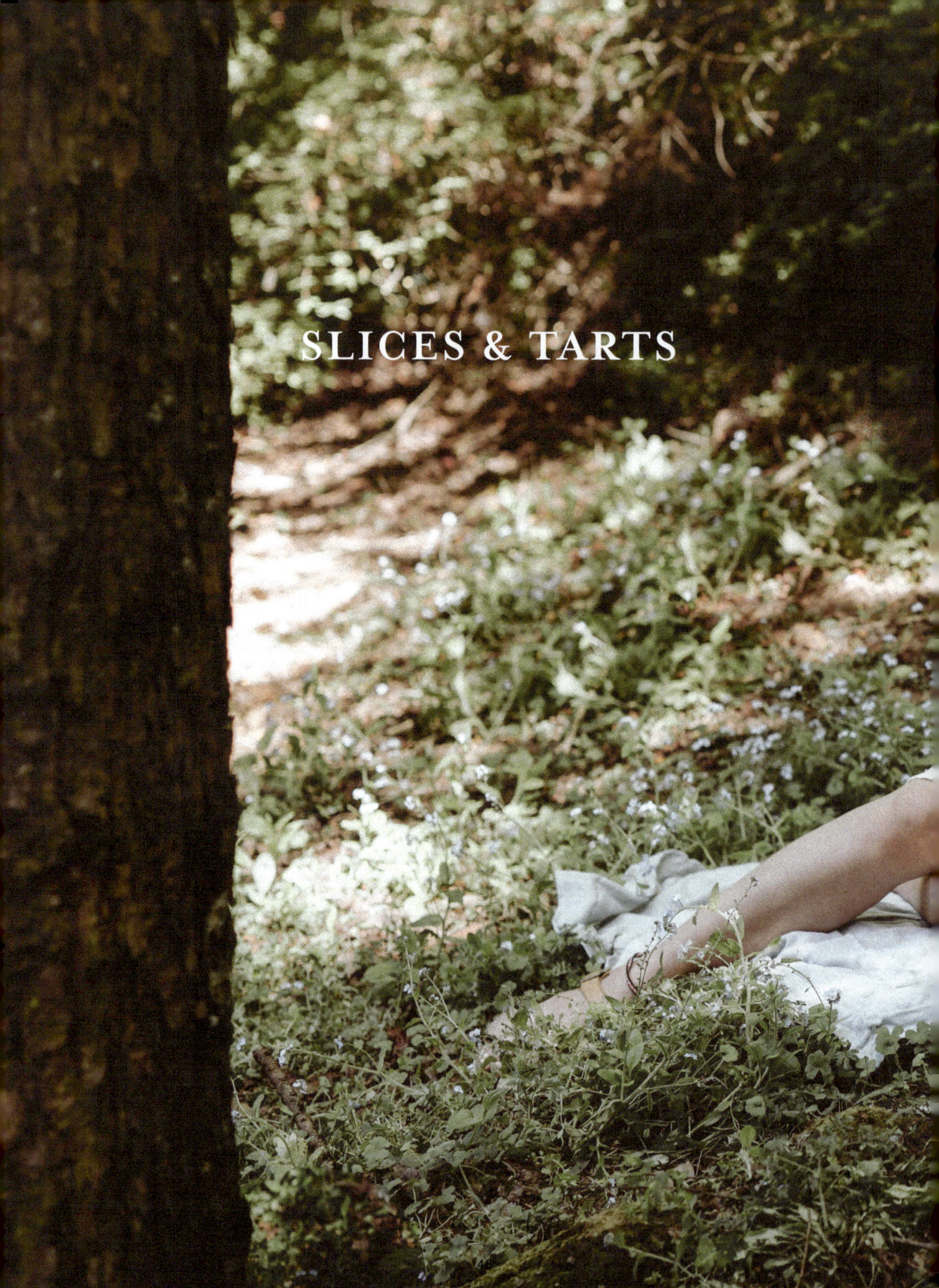

SLICES & TARTS

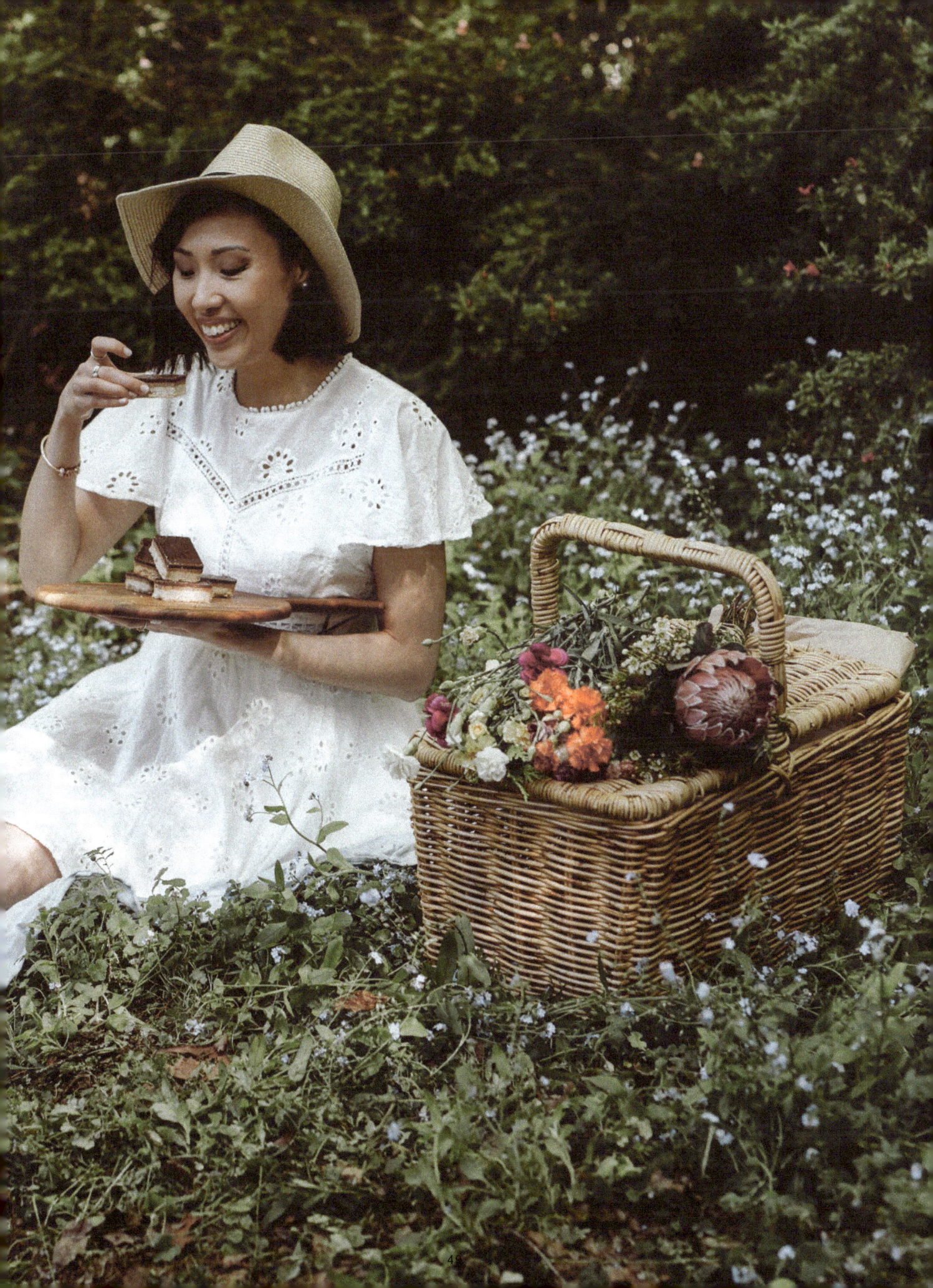

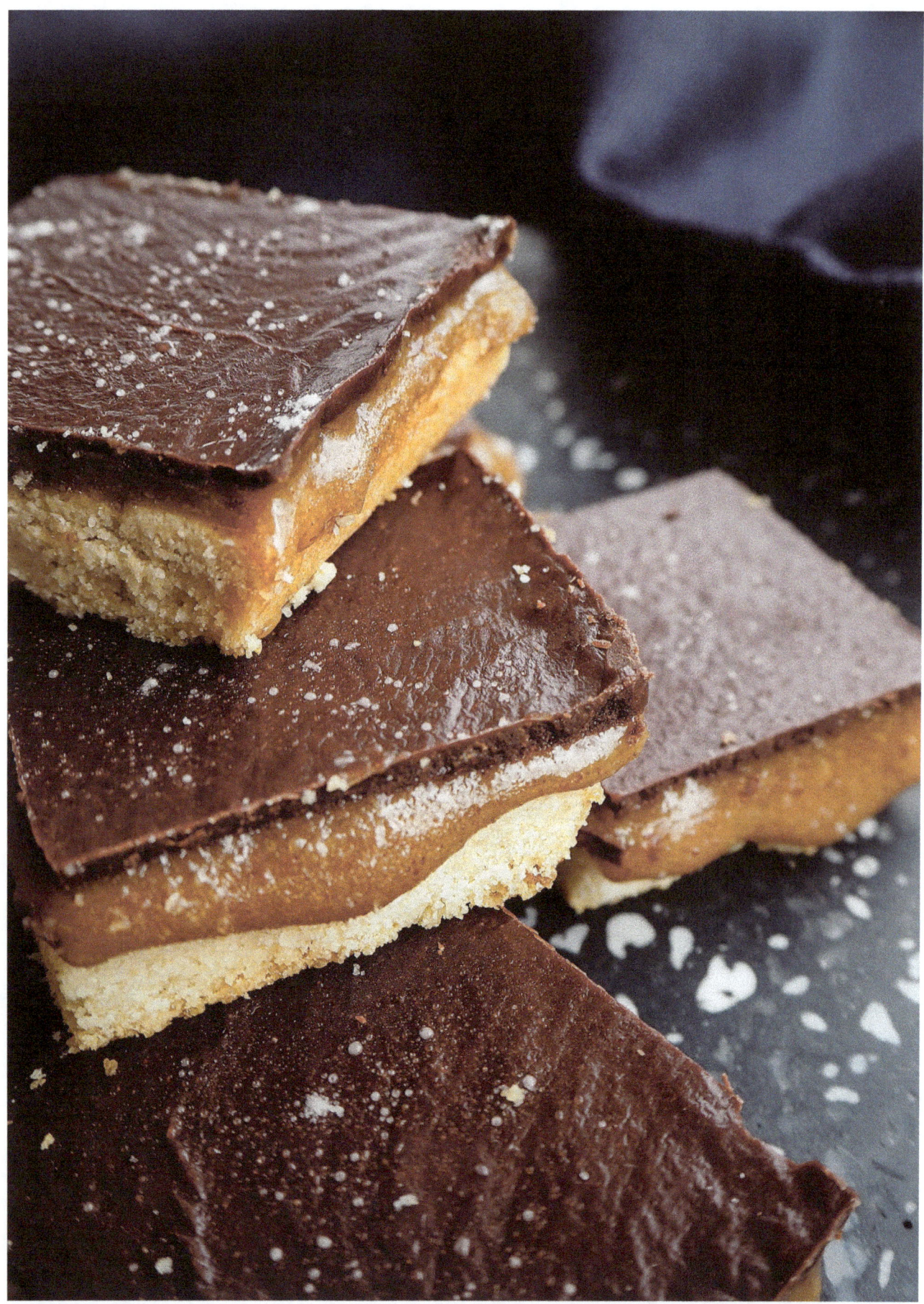

Twist On The Twix

Makes 24 square slices

The Twix is the quintessential combination of a layered biscuit pastry, gooey caramel centre, topped with a delectable chocolate icing — making for a party in your mouth. A tantalising treat for when you are craving something sweet, they are also ideal for making ahead of time to impress guests at your next celebration.

BISCUIT BASE
Refer to Slice and Tart Base — Option 3 on page 87

CARAMEL LAYER
¼ cup smooth almond butter
¼ cup coconut butter, melted
¼ cup pure maple syrup
1 teaspoon pure vanilla extract
2 tablespoons sunflower seed butter
2 tablespoons water
¼ teaspoon salt

CHOCOLATE TOPPING
¼ cup organic extra virgin coconut oil, melted
¼ cup cacao powder
2 tablespoons pure maple syrup
⅛ teaspoon salt
Pinch of cinnamon powder
1 teaspoon pure vanilla extract

Preheat the oven to 180°c and line a 17.5 cm x 27.5 cm slice baking tin. Make the biscuit base by referring to the Slice and Tart Base — Option 3 recipe on page 87.

Once the dough is pressed evenly into the baking tin, use a fork to make holes throughout the base before placing in the oven to bake. This will ensure it does not puff up during the cooking process. Bake for around 20-25 minutes or until lightly browned, turning the tray around at the 10-minute mark. Once cooked, remove and let it cool for 10 minutes in the baking tin, before transferring to a wire rack to cool completely.

While the biscuit base is cooling down, make the caramel layer. In a mixing bowl, whisk all the ingredients together until smooth and creamy. Place the cooled biscuit base back into the baking tin and pour the caramel over it. Refrigerate for 1 hour to set.

Just before the hour is up, make the chocolate topping. In a mixing bowl, combine all ingredients and stir until all of the cacao powder dissolves. Pour the chocolate topping over the hardened caramel layer. Refrigerate for 2 hours until completely set, then slice into 24 squares.

RECIPE NOTES

These Twix slices freeze well. Allow to thaw out for 10-15 minutes before eating, or microwave straight from the freezer for 15 seconds.

Strawberry Jelly Slices

Makes 16 slices

These strawberry jelly slices are simply marvellous. They consist of a decadent vanilla custard sandwiched between a crumbly biscuit base and a refreshing strawberry jelly, infused with mint and basil. Altogether, this makes for a light and delicate slice where the flavours in every layer fuse together in harmony.

BISCUIT BASE
Refer to Slice and Tart Base — Option 1 on page 85, but add the rind of 1 lemon to the dough mix.

VANILLA CUSTARD
1 ½ cups unsweetened almond milk
1 ½ cups organic coconut milk
4 ½ tablespoons tapioca starch
2 teaspoons agar agar flakes
⅓ cup pure maple syrup
1 tablespoon pure vanilla extract (concentrated)
¼ teaspoon salt

STRAWBERRY JELLY LAYER
2 cups organic fresh or frozen strawberries (thaw first before use)
¼ lemon, juiced
3 tablespoons pure maple syrup
1 tablespoon agar agar flakes
½ cup water
Handful of fresh basil and/or mint leaves

Preheat the oven to 200°c and line a 19.5 cm x 29.5 cm slice baking tin. Make the biscuit base by referring to the Slice and Tart Base — Option 1 recipe on page 85.

Once the dough is pressed evenly into the baking tin, use a fork to make holes throughout the base before placing in the oven to bake. This will ensure it does not puff up during the cooking process.

Bake for 20 minutes or until lightly browned, turning the tray around at the 10-minute mark. Once the 20 minutes are up, lower the oven temperature to 175°c and bake for a further 10-15 minutes. Once cooked, remove and let it cool for 10 minutes in the baking tin, before transferring to a wire rack to cool completely.

While the base is cooling down, make the vanilla custard. Pour the almond milk and coconut milk into a saucepan. Add in the tapioca starch and whisk to remove any lumps. On medium heat, add in the maple syrup, vanilla extract, salt and agar agar flakes; whisking frequently until the custard has thickened up nicely. Remove the custard from the stove and cool down for about 10 minutes.

Place the cooled biscuit base back into the baking tin and pour the custard over it, making sure it is even and smooth. Refrigerate for 3 hours to set or leave in the fridge overnight.

After 3 hours or the next day, make the strawberry jelly layer. Process the

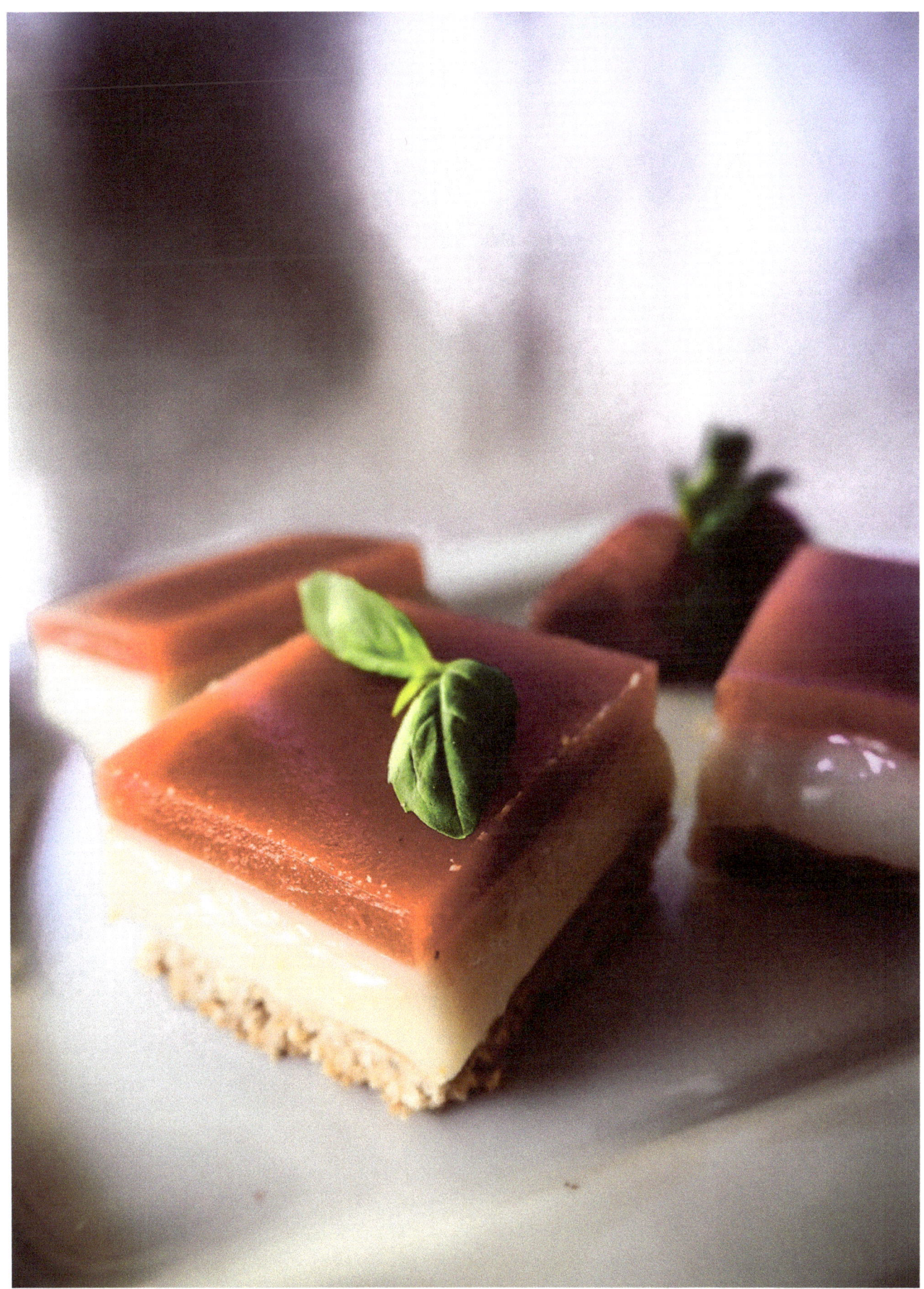

Strawberry Jelly Slices Continued —

strawberries, basil and mint in a food processor or blender until smooth.

Strain the mixture and pour the strawberry liquid into a saucepan. Add in all the other ingredients and bring it to a boil. Simmer for a further 5 minutes, then remove from the heat and allow to cool for 10 minutes.

Remove the chilled slice from the fridge and pour the strawberry jelly over the custard layer. Return to the fridge to chill and set for 2 hours. Slice and serve.

RECIPE NOTES

Once served, store the remaining slices in an airtight container and refrigerate.

This strawberry slice does not freeze well. It is best to store in the fridge for a maximum of 3 days (if it lasts that long!).

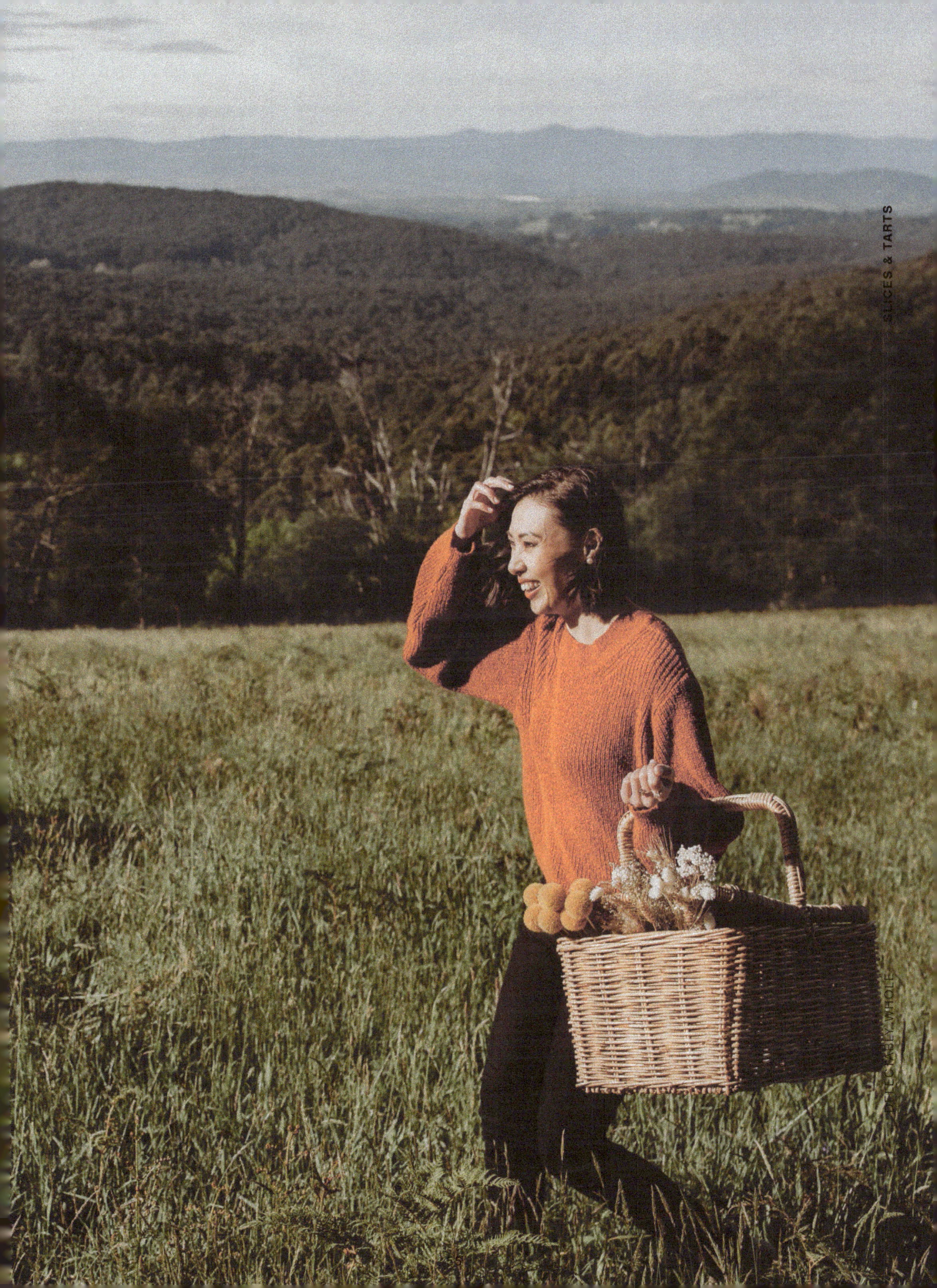

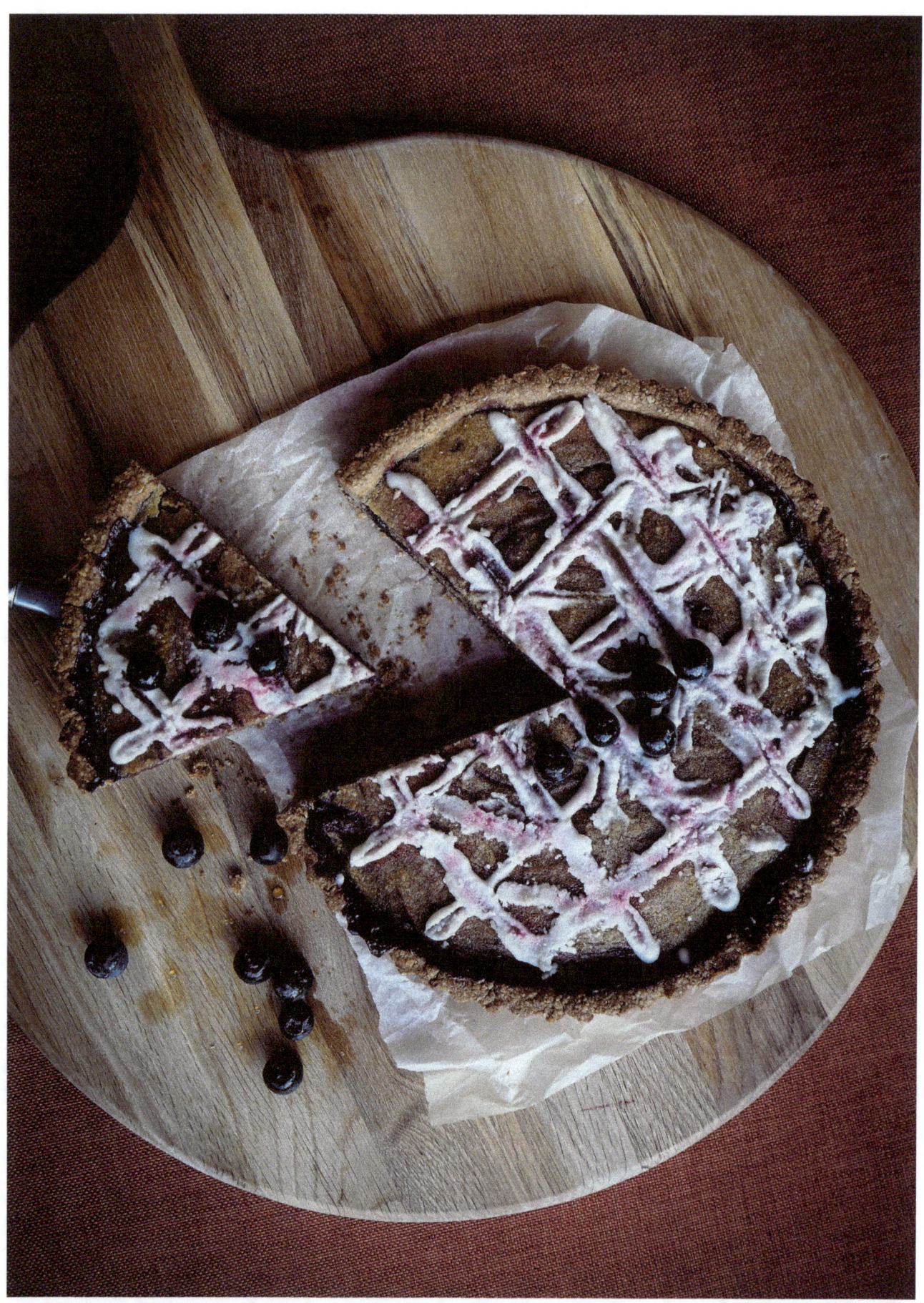

Blueberry Frangipane Tart

Makes 12 to 20 slices

This tart is a real winner! A luscious blueberry jam layer encased in a crispy and oaty biscuit pastry, topped with a soft-baked almond-flavoured custard. A perfect autumn or winter dessert, it is best served warm with some coconut ice-cream.

TART PASTRY
Refer to Slice and Tart base — Option 1 on page 85

BERRY LAYER
1 ½ cups fresh/frozen organic blueberries
½ cup water
2 teaspoons lemon juice
Zest of ½ lemon
2 tablespoons pure maple syrup
1 tablespoon tapioca starch
½ teaspoon pure vanilla extract
Pinch of salt

FRANGIPANE TOPPING
½ cup sorghum flour or chestnut flour
½ cup blended pecans, fine
¼ cup organic extra virgin coconut oil, melted
3 tablespoons pure maple syrup
1 free-range egg
1 free-range egg yolk
1 teaspoon pure vanilla extract
Pinch of salt
½ teaspoon pure almond essence
Zest of ½ lemon

Preheat the oven to 200°c. Grease either a round 25 cm tart tin with removable base or a 21.5 cm x 31 cm tart tin. Set aside.

Make the tart pastry by referring to the Slice and Tart Base — Option 1 recipe on page 85.

Once the dough is pressed evenly into the baking tin, use a fork to make holes throughout the base before placing in the oven to bake. Blind bake the tart case for 20 minutes.

While the tart is baking, make the blueberry filling by placing all the ingredients into a saucepan and bringing it to a boil, stirring frequently. Then, lower to a gentle simmer until it thickens and let it cool.

Make the frangipane topping by whisking together all the ingredients until smooth. Once the tart is out of the oven, pour the blueberry filling into the tart shell.

Spoon the frangipane mixture on top of the blueberry filling, making sure to cover the blueberries along the sides, to avoid it bubbling over. As an option, you can gently stir through the top to create a swirl effect.

Lower the oven temperature to 170°c and bake the tart for 40 minutes. Let it cool and place it in the fridge to set for 2 hours before serving.

RECIPE NOTES

This tart freezes well. Freeze tart slices in an airtight container. To reheat from frozen, bake the tart at 165°c for 15 minutes and serve.

Pecan Tart

Makes 12 slices

What is there not to love about a pecan tart? Exquisitely decadent and perfectly sweet, the hero of this tart is the wonderful caramelisation of the toasted pecans smothered in maple, combined with the addition of creamy yam, which complements the nuttiness and adds a unique depth of flavour. A crispy shortcrust pastry encases all of this, making it ideal with a dollop of coconut ice-cream and a hot cuppa.

TART PASTRY
Refer to Slice and Tart Base — Option 2 on page 86

FILLING
¾ cup pure maple syrup
⅓ cup coconut sugar
2 free-range eggs, beaten
2 tablespoons organic extra virgin coconut oil, melted
2 tablespoons sunflower seed butter
2 teaspoons pure vanilla extract
1 cup packed, cooked mashed purple yam
¼ teaspoon salt
1 cup pecans (chopped) plus extra for decorating

Preheat the oven to 190°c. Grease a round 25 cm tart tin with a removable base and set aside.

Make the tart pastry by referring to the Slice and Tart Base — Option 2 recipe on page 86.

While the dough is resting in the fridge, cook the yam. Peel a medium-sized yam and cut away the hard outer layer. Slice it into small pieces and place into a large saucepan or stainless steel frying pan. Set aside 1 cup of water, and pour some in with the yam pieces, cover and let steam on medium to low heat. The yam will absorb the liquid quite quickly, so be sure to check it often, adding more water as it cooks until all the water is absorbed.

Mash the yam pieces with a fork to break it down. Then, using a wooden spoon, stir vigorously until it becomes a thick sticky paste. Preparing and cooking the yam will take roughly 15 to 20 minutes. Once cooked, set aside to cool (it will harden as it cools).

Once the dough is pressed evenly into the baking tin, use a fork to make holes throughout the base before placing in the oven to bake. Blind bake the pie shell for 15 minutes. Remove and let it cool.

While the tart shell is baking, make the pecan filling by mixing all ingredients in a bowl, until well incorporated.

Turn the oven temperature down to 175°c. Once the tart shell has cooled slightly, pour the pecan filling into the shell and bake for 45 minutes.

Remove and allow the tart to cool down. Then, place it in the fridge to set for at least 2 hours before serving.

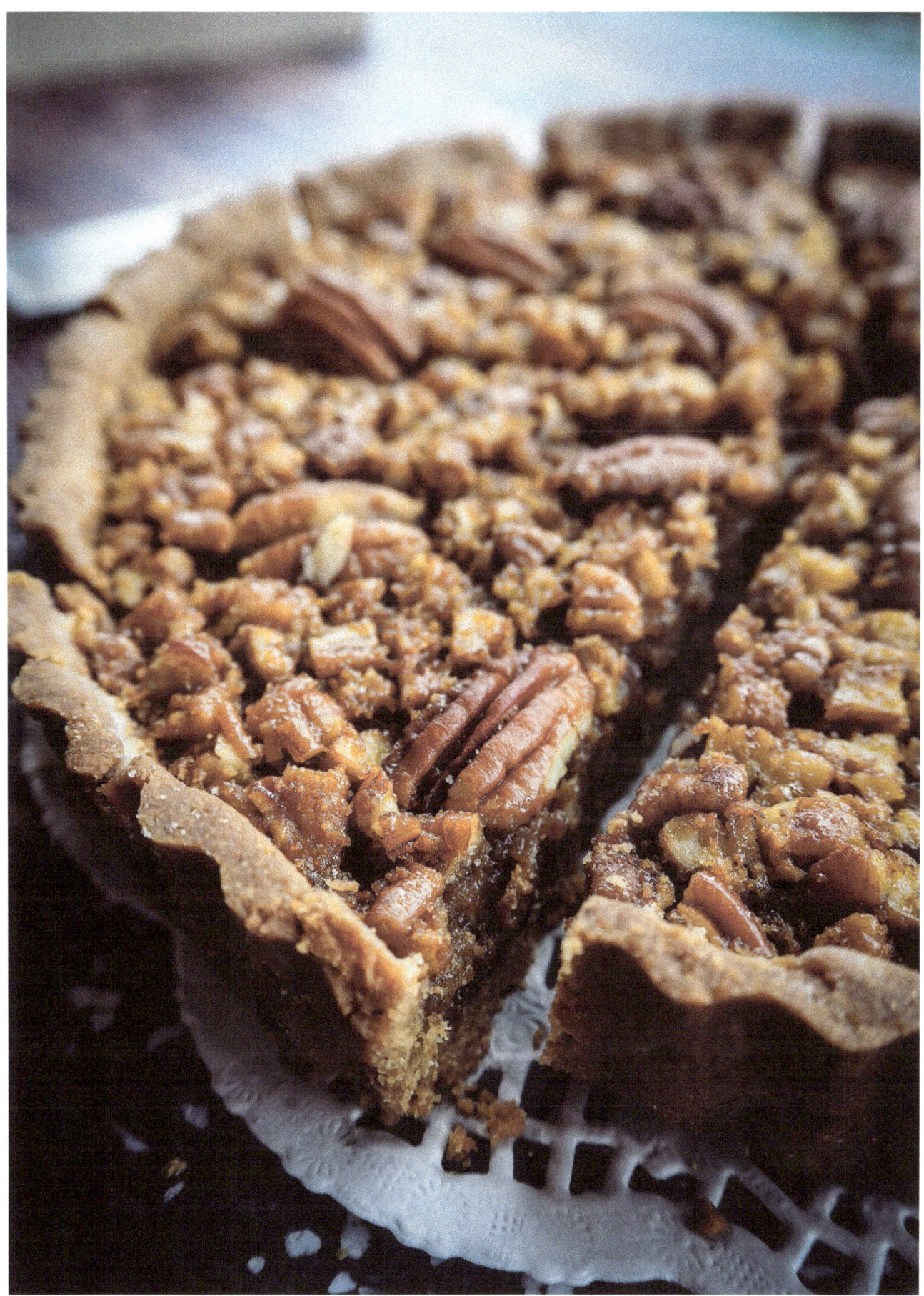

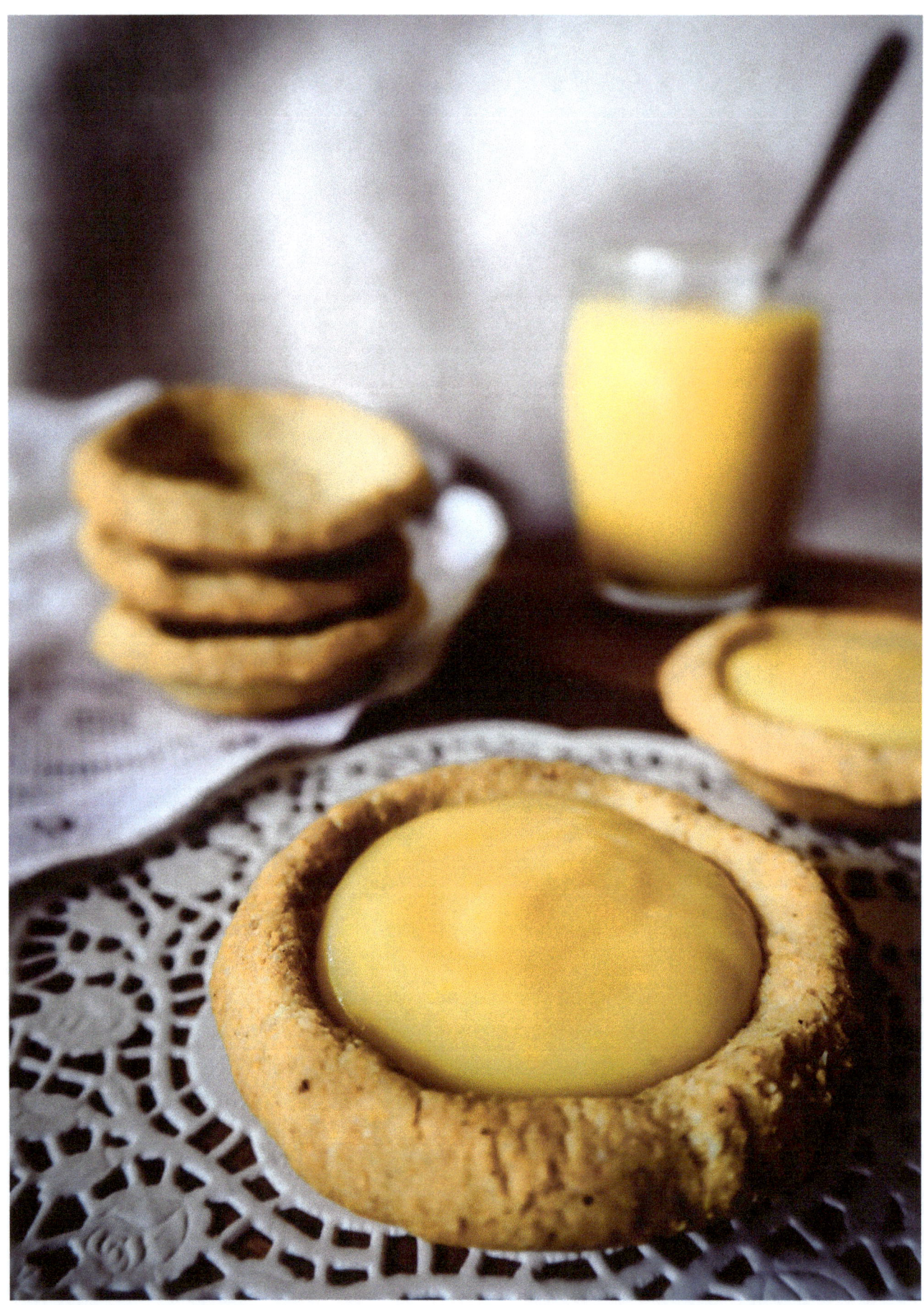

Lemon Curd Tartlets

Curd makes 2 medium-sized jars
Tart pastry makes 18 mini tartlet shells

If you are a fan of good lemon curd, this one will not disappoint. This luscious lemon curd balances the tartness and sweetness exquisitely and together with the crunchy shortbread crust, your mouth will be exploding with zesty and crumbly goodness.

LEMON CURD
3 free-range eggs
½ cup fresh lemon juice (2 medium lemons)
1 tablespoon grated lemon zest
½ cup pure maple syrup
½ cup organic extra virgin coconut oil, melted
¼ teaspoon salt
1 teaspoon pure vanilla extract
1 tablespoon arrowroot starch

TARTLET SHELLS
Refer to Slice and Tart Base — Option 3 on page 87. Add 1 tablespoon of golden flaxseed meal to the dough mix.

In a saucepan, whisk together the eggs, lemon juice, lemon zest, maple syrup, vanilla extract, salt and arrowroot starch. Heat the mixture on medium heat, whisking for about 1 to 2 minutes until all combined, then whisk frequently. Once it starts to thicken, add the melted coconut oil and whisk on medium-low heat for another 2-3 minutes until creamy and thick.

Remove from the heat and pour the curd through a fine mesh strainer into a glass bowl (using a spatula to do so). Cool the curd until it becomes room temperature and place in the fridge to set.

Preheat the oven to 180°c. While the curd is cooling down, make the tartlet shells by referring to the Slice and Tart Base — Option 3 recipe on page 87.

Spoon 1.5 teaspoon-sized balls into a 12-hole, 6 cm-diameter mini tart tray (with inbuilt holes at the bottom of each mould), or 1.5 tablespoon-sized balls if using a standard muffin tray. Mould each ball into the shape of the tartlet mould, so that all the sides and bottoms are equal in thickness. Using a fork, poke holes into the base of the dough in each tartlet mould. This will prevent the base of the tartlets from rising and the sides from sinking.

Bake for 20-25 minutes until golden and cooked through, turning the tray around after 12 minutes of baking. Once cooked, remove the tray from the oven and let the tartlets cool in their moulds for 5 minutes. Then, slowly and gently ease each tartlet out from their moulds, taking great care not to break them. If they do not remove easily, gently scrape the bottoms of the tart tray (as the baked dough seeps through the inbuilt holes and seals the tartlets in). This should make it easier to remove the tartlets. Place them on a cooling rack to cool completely.

Spoon the cold lemon curd into each tartlet and serve.

RECIPE NOTES

The lemon curd will last for about 5 days in the fridge. Alternatively, you can freeze the curd in portions, using an ice-cube tray and defrost it in the fridge until ready to eat. The tartlet shells can be frozen in an airtight container and defrosted to room temperature 10 minutes before serving. Only spoon the curd into the tartlet shells just before eating, as the curd will soften the shells if they are stored together for a long time.

Baked Oat Granola Bars

Makes 12 bars

Soft, chewy and simply delicious, these baked oat granola bars are chock-full of wholesome and nutritious ingredients. Enjoy them for breakfast on-the-go, as post-workout munchies or as a special treat in the kids' lunchboxes.

¼ cup organic extra virgin coconut oil, melted
¼ cup pure maple syrup
1 teaspoon pure vanilla extract
1 tablespoon tahini, hulled
1 tablespoon sunflower seed butter
¼ cup coconut sugar
1 free-range egg
¼ cup unsweetened almond milk
½ cup rolled oats
¼ cup oat flour
¼ cup Gluten-Free Flour Blend — Option 2
¼ cup desiccated coconut
2 cups mixed puff cereal (brown rice puffs, sorghum puffs, quinoa puffs, millet puffs, buckwheat puffs)
1 cup mixed nuts (pecans, macadamias, brazil nuts, almonds, hazelnuts)
¼ cup of pepitas and sunflower seeds mix
1 tablespoon golden flaxseed meal
1 tablespoon hemp flour
¼ cup dried cranberries
½ teaspoon cinnamon powder
¼ teaspoon salt
¼ teaspoon baking soda

Preheat the oven to 180°c and line a 17.5 cm x 27.5 cm brownie tin. In a food processor, blitz together the mixed puff cereal, nuts and dried cranberries until finely grounded.

In a bowl, mix together maple syrup, coconut sugar, coconut oil, tahini, sunflower seed butter, vanilla extract, coconut sugar, egg, almond milk, cinnamon powder, salt and baking soda until well combined.

Stir in the nut and cereal mix, along with the rolled oats, oat flour, desiccated coconut, seeds, flaxseed meal, and flours with the wet ingredients until it becomes a sticky consistency.

Press firmly to flatten into the brownie tin. Bake at 180°c for 25 minutes. Let it cool before slicing into bars.

RECIPE NOTES

Store bars in an airtight container in the fridge if eating daily.

To freeze, wrap bars in baking paper and cling wrap, and place in an airtight container. Bring them to room temperature before eating, or warm them up in the microwave for 40 seconds.

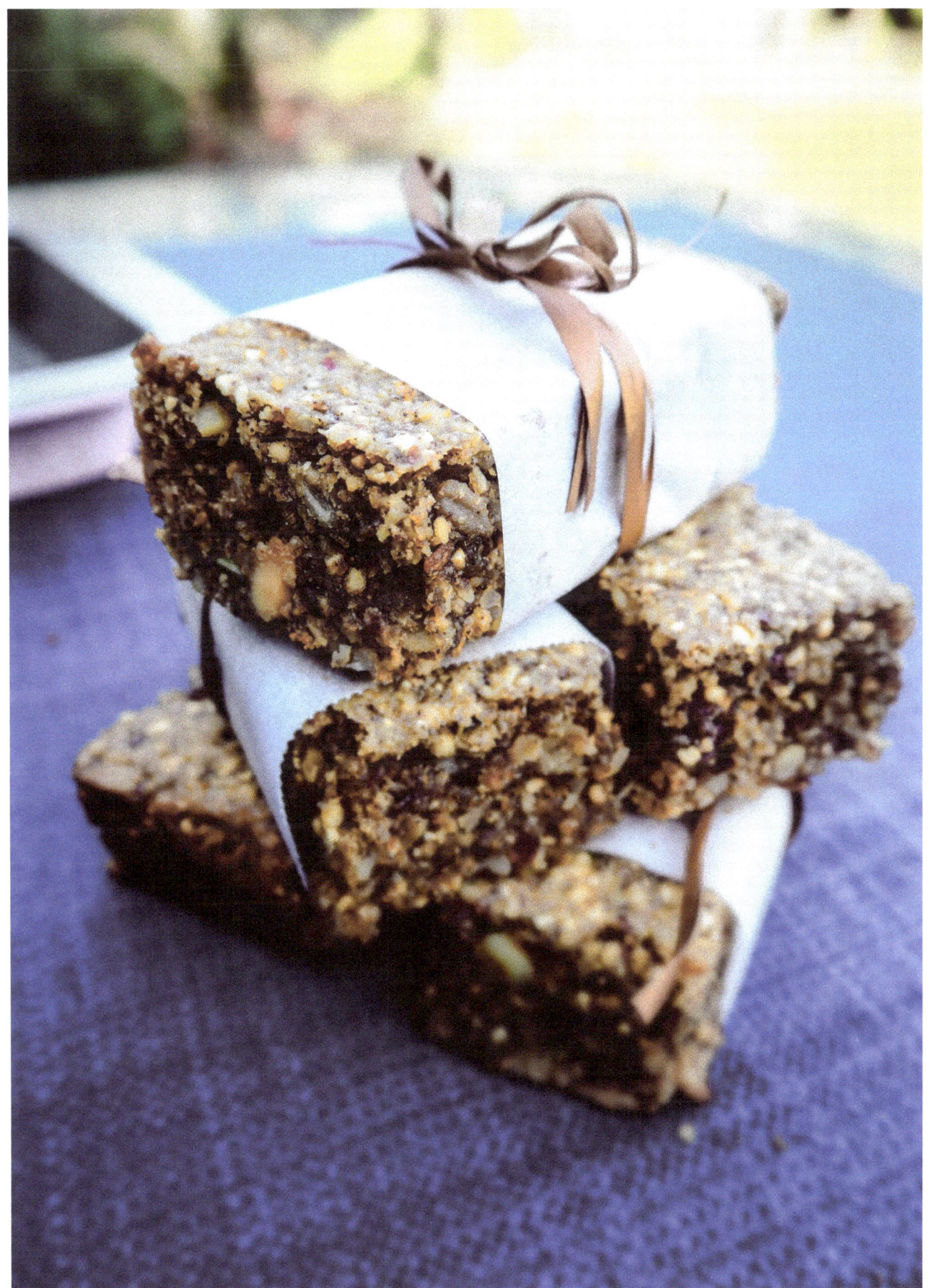

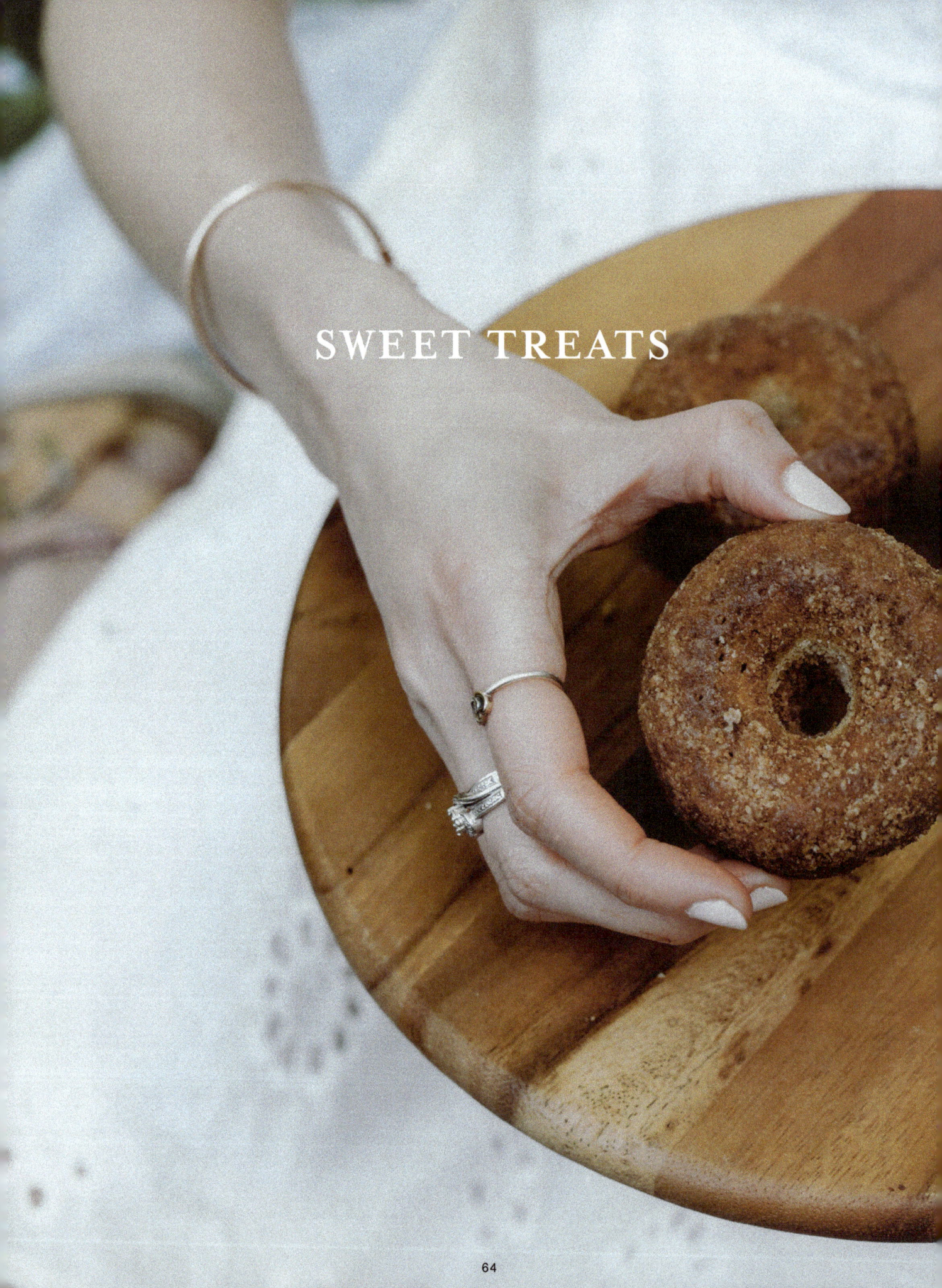

SWEET TREATS

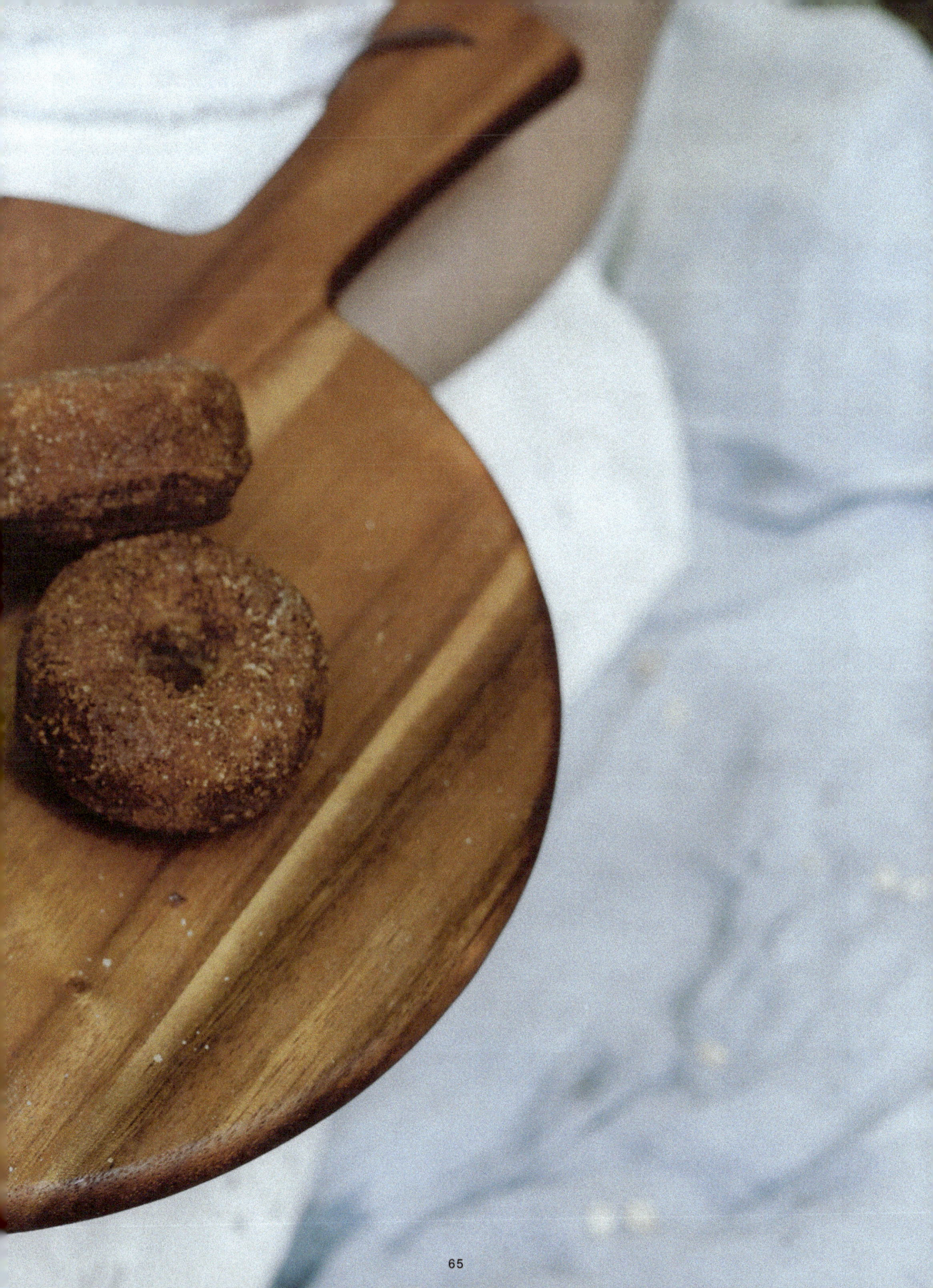

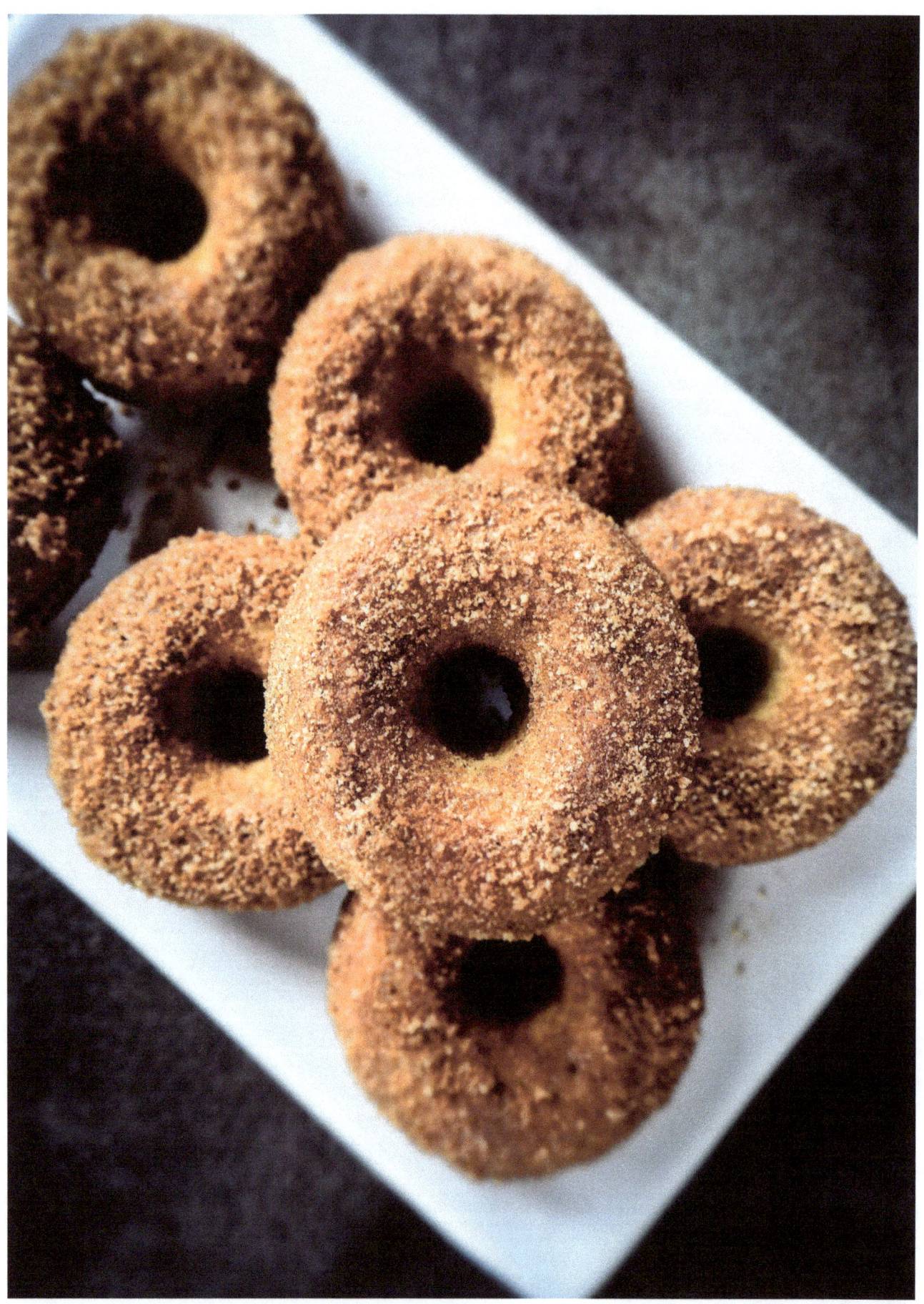

Cinnamon Doughnuts

Makes between 11-14 doughnuts

These joy-inducing goodies are nicknamed 'Dynamic Doughnuts' by my 'bestie', and I've got to tell you, they are definitely worth celebrating! Forget about the deep-fried sugary equivalents — these will change your mind on baked doughnuts forever. You will remember these by their beautifully crisp, sweet outer, and their soft and fluffy insides. Here's to enjoying many more doughnuts — guilt-free!

½ cup sorghum flour
½ cup blanched almond flour
¼ cup coconut flour
¼ cup tapioca starch or arrowroot starch
4 tablespoons potato starch
2 tablespoons glutinous rice flour
¼ cup pure maple syrup
1 teaspoon baking powder
½ teaspoon baking soda
¼ teaspoon salt
¼ cup olive oil or organic extra virgin coconut oil, melted
¾ cup unsweetened almond milk
3 free-range eggs
½ teaspoon apple cider vinegar
¼ teaspoon cinnamon powder
2 teaspoons pure vanilla extract

SUGAR COATING
2 tablespoons vegan butter (melted) or organic extra virgin coconut oil for brushing the doughnuts
⅓ cup coconut sugar and maple sugar mix
1 ½ teaspoons cinnamon powder
⅛ teaspoon salt

Preheat the oven to 175°c. In a mixing bowl, whisk together the olive oil or coconut oil, eggs, maple syrup, vanilla extract, apple cider vinegar and almond milk together until combined. Add in the flours, baking powder, baking soda, salt and cinnamon powder and whisk until a smooth batter is formed.

Pour the batter into two greased 7 cm or 8 cm 6-mould doughnut tins, filling each mould three quarters of the way. Bake the doughnuts for 25 minutes, until golden brown.

When the doughnuts are completely cool, remove them from the moulds and brush each one with oil on both sides. In a bowl, mix together the sugar coating until thoroughly combined. Lightly toss the doughnuts in the sugar coating until evenly coated on all sides. Eat immediately or store in an airtight container.

RECIPE NOTES

These doughnuts can be kept in the fridge for 3-4 days or in the freezer for 1 month. To reheat frozen doughnuts, bake at 175°c for 10 minutes. Once they cool down for 5-10 minutes, they are extra crispy on the outside, but still soft and fluffy on the inside.

Banana Pancakes

Makes 8 medium-sized pancakes

One of my favourite breakfast treats is banana pancakes! For me, they have to be light, fluffy, moist and beautifully golden brown. These are absolutely scrumptious and best of all, you can substitute whatever flours you have in your pantry that morning. I love to drizzle my pancakes with maple syrup, topped with fresh blueberries. If you are in the mood for something a little more savoury, pair them with caramelised maple bacon and a sunny side-up egg. Your options are endless!

½ cup oat flour or toasted quinoa flour
¼ cup sorghum flour or teff flour
¼ cup brown rice flour or millet flour

These flour options work well, too:
½ cup oat flour & ½ cup teff flour
OR
½ cup oat flour & ½ cup tiger nut flour
OR
½ cup oat flour & ½ cup millet flour

1 teaspoon baking powder
1 free-range egg
1 cup unsweetened almond milk
2-3 medium-sized ripe bananas
Pinch of salt
Pinch of cinnamon
1 teaspoon pure vanilla extract
Blueberries (optional)

Mix all ingredients together in a mixing bowl.

Drizzle some oil in a non-stick frying pan and wait for the oil to heat up. Over low-medium heat, spoon 1 or 2 ladles of batter into the pan.

Once bubbles start to form on the surface, flip the pancakes over, leaving them approximately 2 minutes on each side, or until golden brown.

Serve them up warm.

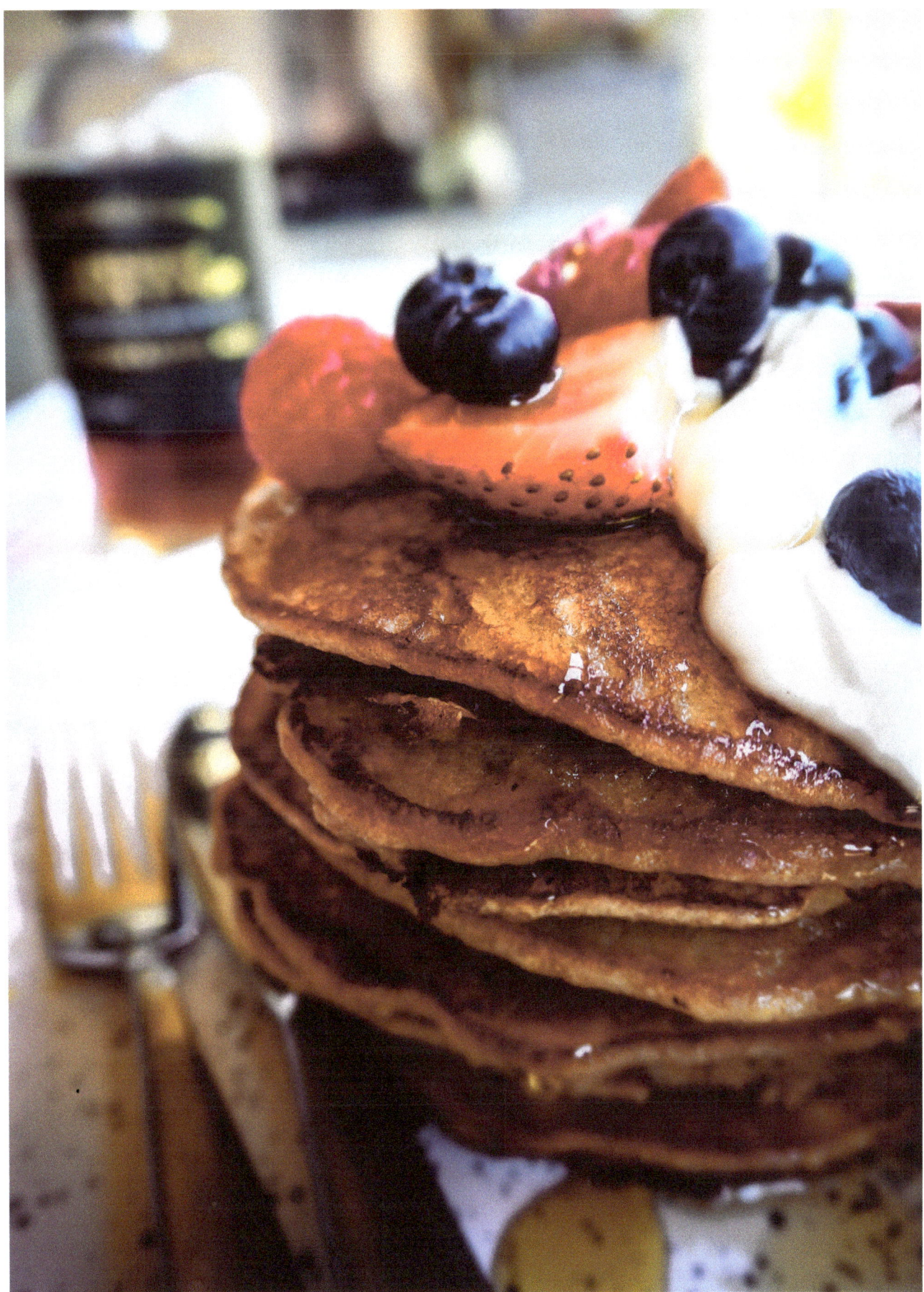

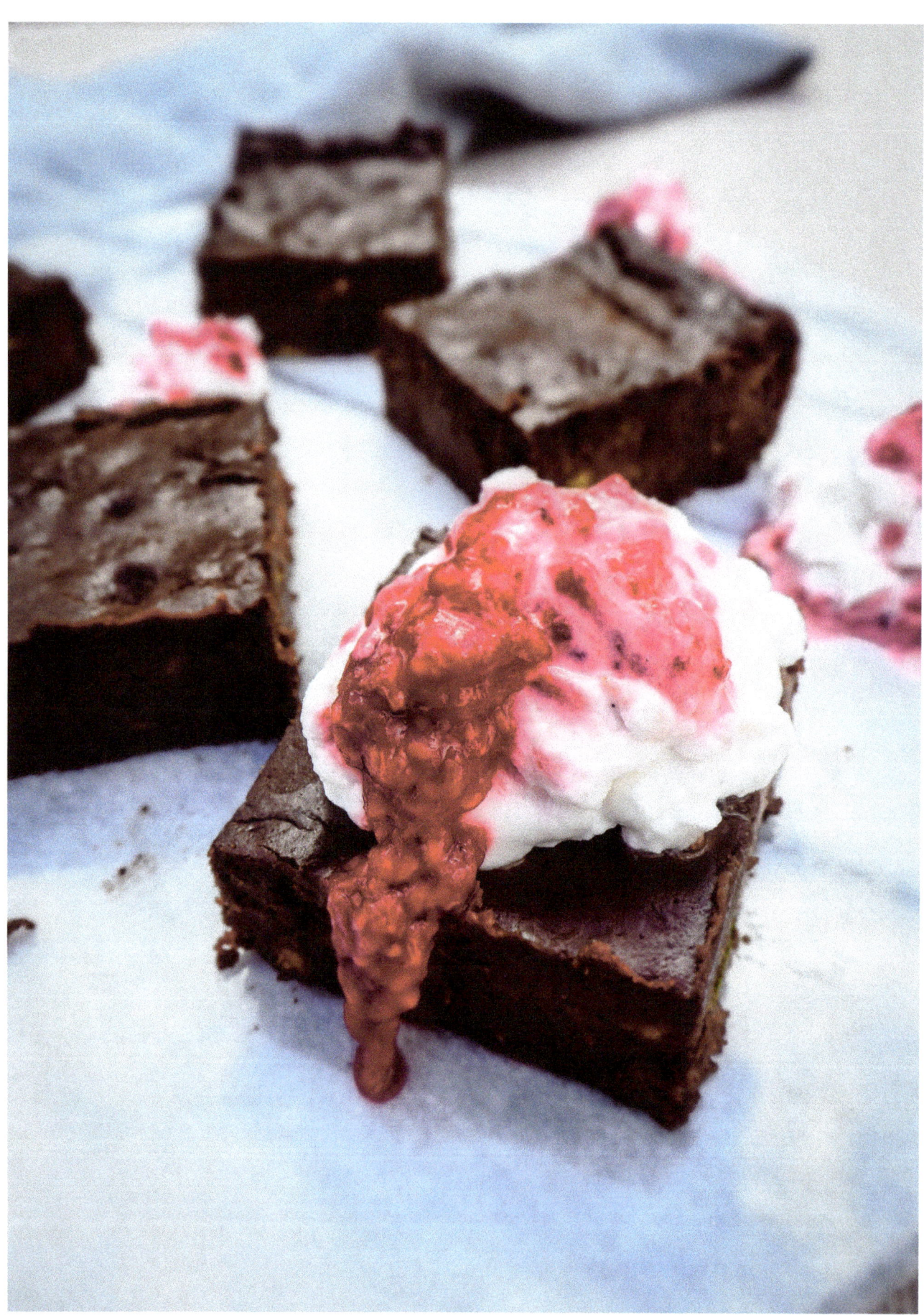

Fudgy Chocolate Brownies

Makes 15 slices

All you chocolate-lovers out there — this brownie is for you! Decadently rich and fudgy, it just melts in your mouth. Best of all, it contains fibre and nutrient-rich vegetables like sweet potato and zucchini, plus antioxidants from the cacao and dark chocolate. A little goes a long way to satisfy any sweet tooth, and pairs perfectly with coconut vanilla ice cream, yoghurt, or topped with raspberries for a special healthy treat.

2 free-range eggs
¼ cup pure maple syrup
¼ cup coconut sugar
¼ cup organic extra virgin coconut oil, melted
½ cup heaped sweet potato puree
1 medium zucchini, grated and juice squeezed
½ cup unsweetened coconut yoghurt or applesauce
1 teaspoon pure vanilla extract
90 g of 70% or 85% dark chocolate, melted
¼ cup cacao powder
¼ cup smooth almond butter or sunflower seed butter
2 tablespoons sorghum, hemp or teff flour
½ teaspoon baking soda
½ teaspoon salt
¼ cup dark chocolate chips or 45 g of 70% dark chocolate, chopped coarsely
¼ teaspoon cinnamon powder
50 ml freshly brewed decaffeinated coffee (or regular coffee, if preferred)

Preheat the oven to 175°c. Steam roughly half a sweet potato and mash to produce ½ a cup of sweet potato puree.

In a mixing bowl, melt the coconut oil and whisk in maple syrup, coconut sugar, eggs and vanilla until combined. Add in the sweet potato puree, grated zucchini, coconut yoghurt, melted dark chocolate, almond or sunflower seed butter and coffee. Whisk well until smooth.

Add in cacao powder, flour, baking soda, cinnamon and salt, then stir with a spatula or wooden spoon. Stir in the chocolate chips or chopped dark chocolate through until just combined.

Pour batter into a lined 19.5 cm x 29.5 cm brownie tin and smooth the top. Bake in the oven for 20 minutes, then turn the tray around and lower the oven temperature to 160°c, baking for a further 10 minutes. Remove from the oven once the middle is just set but still slightly wobbly. Let it cool completely, then keep in the fridge for 2 hours to set before slicing.

RECIPE NOTES

Brownies become fudgier when stored in the fridge. They are also freezer-friendly and can be stored in an airtight container.

To reheat from frozen, let it defrost until room temperature or microwave for 30 seconds.

Tiramisu

Serves 10 people

Tiramisu has got to be one of my all-time favourite desserts and has become somewhat of a Christmas dessert tradition in my family. The fusion of coffee and liquor-soaked Savoiardi biscuits with the creaminess of the mascarpone is just out of this world. I have revamped this classic recipe to produce a dairy-free, non-alcoholic, histamine and child-friendly version that the whole family can enjoy. The blend of pomegranate, chocolate and coffee create depth and complexity in place of the liquor, without compromising on flavour, resulting in a deliciously decadent dessert!

SAVOIARDI BISCUITS
MAKES 24
½ cup almond flour
¼ cup brown rice flour
¼ cup tapioca or arrowroot starch
1 teaspoon baking powder
¼ teaspoon salt
1 teaspoon pure vanilla extract
4 free-range egg whites, room temperature
3 free-range egg yolks
⅓ cup maple sugar
Coconut flower nectar sugar for sprinkling on top

DAIRY-FREE 'MASCARPONE' — OPTION 1 (if you prefer a cream-based texture)
2 x 400 g cans of coconut cream
1 teaspoon lemon juice
¼ cup maple sugar
2 teaspoons pure vanilla extract

DAIRY FREE 'MASCARPONE' — OPTION 2 (if you prefer a custard-like texture)
1 ½ cups unsweetened almond milk
1 cup coconut milk
1 teaspoon lemon juice
⅓ cup maple sugar
2 teaspoons pure vanilla extract
¼ teaspoon pure almond extract
¼ teaspoon salt
¼ cup arrowroot starch

Preheat the oven to 180°C. In a bowl, combine the almond flour, brown rice flour, tapioca starch, baking powder and salt together.

In a separate bowl, beat the egg whites with 1 tablespoon of the maple sugar until stiff peaks form.

In another bowl, whisk together the egg yolks, vanilla extract and the remaining maple sugar until creamy. Gently fold the egg whites into the egg yolk mixture, followed by the dry ingredients until combined.

Pour the mixture into a piping bag and pipe 4 x 8 cm lady-finger shapes onto a lined baking tray, making sure there are 24 of them all together.

Lightly sprinkle some coconut flower nectar sugar on top of each biscuit and bake for 13 minutes, then reduce the oven temperature to 160°C and bake for a further 15 minutes to harden slightly.

Remove and let them cool on a cooling rack.

DAIRY-FREE 'MASCARPONE' — OPTION 1
Refrigerate both cans of coconut cream overnight. This will split the liquid part from the hardened cream. The following day, pour the hardened cream only (not the liquid part) into a bowl. Save the liquid part for curries or smoothies. Add the lemon juice, maple sugar and vanilla extract and whip the cream until it is smooth, light and fluffy. Refrigerate until it is ready to use.

DAIRY-FREE 'MASCARPONE' — OPTION 2
Place all of the ingredients into a saucepan and heat on medium heat, stirring frequently until the mixture thickens and becomes creamy and smooth. Remove from heat and let it cool completely.

I like to place it in the fridge to cool for a few hours before I assemble the tiramisu. Before assembling, whisk the custard (as it would have set) to create a creamy smooth texture once again.

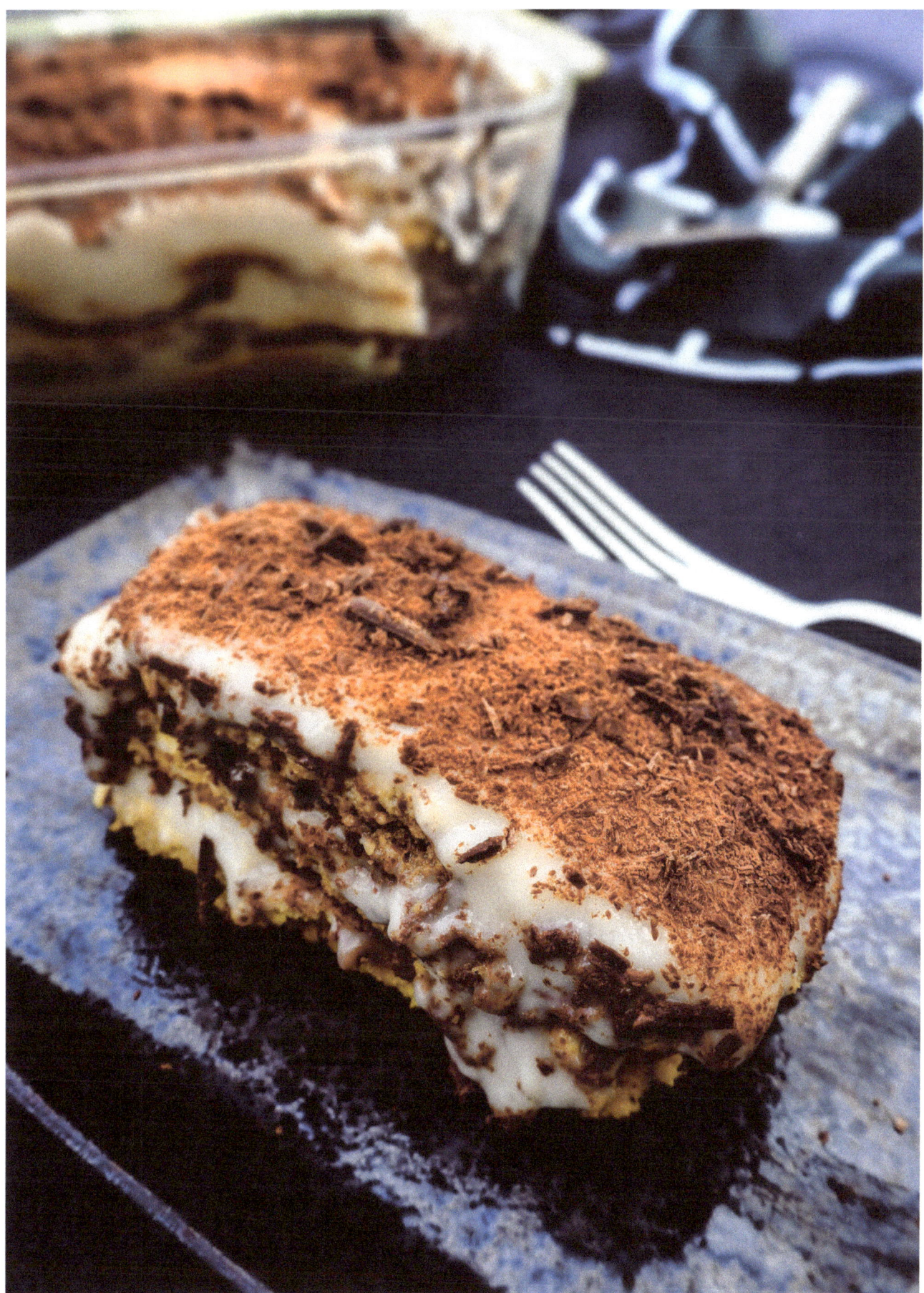

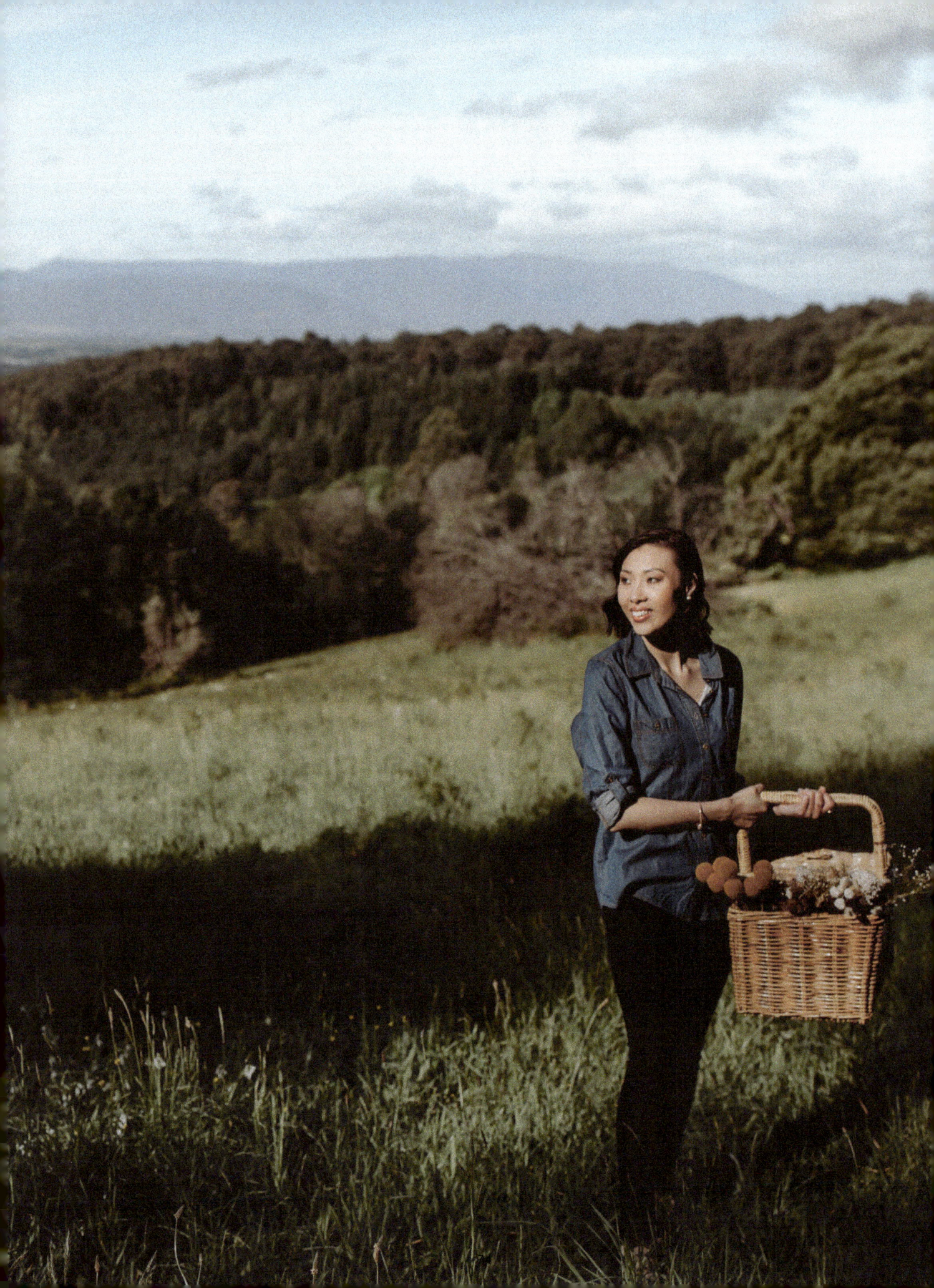

COFFEE AND POMEGRANATE MIXTURE
200 ml freshly brewed decaffeinated coffee (or regular coffee, if preferred)
120 ml pure pomegranate juice
3 tablespoons coconut sugar

Cacao powder for dusting
90g 70% dark chocolate, grated

ASSEMBLING

You will need a 21 cm x 21 cm dish (this will create 3 layers) or a 19 cm x 28 cm dish (2 layers) to assemble the tiramisu in. This recipe features 3 layers.

In a coffee plunger, mix 2 tablespoons of coffee grounds in hot water. Let it sit for about 5 minutes, then pour into a glass measuring jug. Top it off with more hot water to produce 200 ml of liquid. Add the pomegranate juice and coconut sugar to the hot liquid and stir to combine. Set aside.

Having all the elements ready and prepared, start by dunking each Savoiardi biscuit into the coffee pomegranate mixture, turning each about 4 times before lining 8 Savoiardi biscuits on the bottom of the dish in the same formation. Spoon a third of the cream or custard on top, spreading it out evenly. Dust with cacao powder, then sprinkle a third of the grated dark chocolate evenly.

Repeat this process with the next layer, this time laying the Savoiardi biscuits in the opposite formation as the previous layer (in a criss-cross pattern). This will provide stability and structure when cutting through and serving.

Repeat this process for the third time, and pour over any remaining coffee pomegranate mixture over the biscuit layers so they soak through. Finish off the assembly with the remaining cream or custard on top, followed by a dusting of cacao powder and grated chocolate on top.

Cling wrap the dish and place in the fridge to set overnight.

RECIPE NOTES

If histamines are not an issue for you, you can use the traditional masala liquor instead of the pomegranate juice, and omit the coconut sugar, as the liquor is sweet enough.

Tiramisu lasts for about 3-4 days in the fridge and tastes even better from day 2, as all the flavours have time to soak and infuse together.

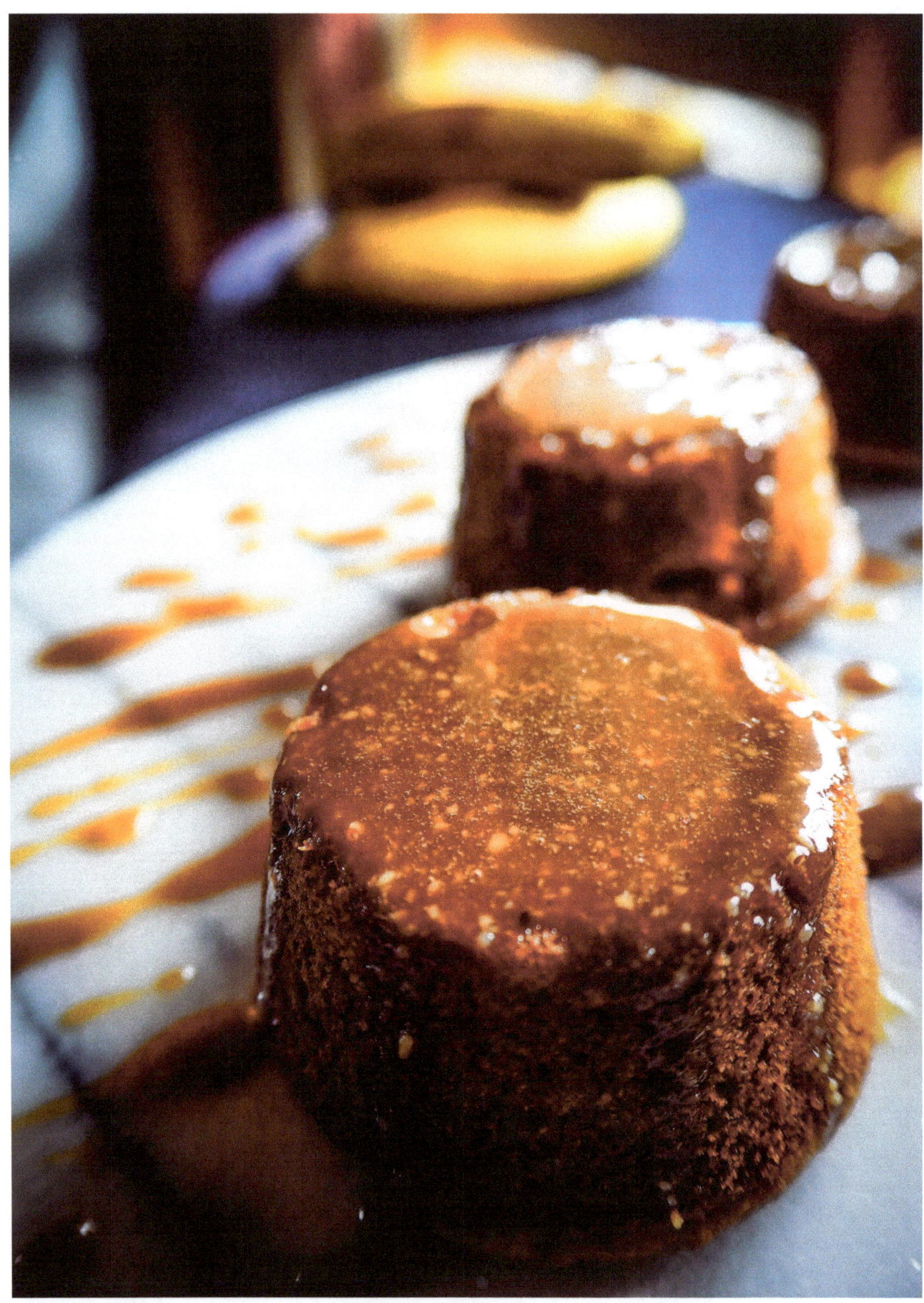

Sticky Banana Puddings with Caramel Sauce

Makes 16 standard puddings

These banana puddings are reminiscent of a traditional sticky date pudding — without the dates! Warm, super moist, sweet and sticky with a nutty caramelised flavour; they are simply scrumptious. This is such a great dessert to make when entertaining family or friends, or just to treat yourself with.

⅓ cup organic extra virgin coconut oil, melted
¼ cup pure maple syrup
2 free-range eggs
4 medium-sized bananas
1 cup unsweetened coconut yoghurt
1 teaspoon pure vanilla extract
½ teaspoon apple cider vinegar
1 teaspoon baking powder
½ teaspoon baking soda
¼ teaspoon salt
¼ teaspoon cinnamon powder
A handful of pecans (optional)
¼ cup brown rice flour
¼ cup millet flour
¼ cup tapioca starch
½ cup oat flour
¼ cup sorghum flour or teff flour or toasted quinoa flour
¼ cup almond flour or tiger nut flour for a nut-free version

CARAMEL SAUCE (FOR DRIZZLING ON TOP)
See Caramel Sauce recipe on page 104

Preheat the oven to 180°c and grease two 12-hole muffin tins, unlined.

Whisk coconut oil, maple syrup and eggs together until smooth. Add in mashed bananas, coconut yoghurt, cinnamon powder, vanilla extract, salt, baking powder, baking soda and apple cider vinegar. Whisk well.

Add in the gluten-free flours and stir until just combined.

Place a pecan at the bottom of each muffin hole. Pour the muffin batter into each hole until just full, covering the pecans. Bake for 30 minutes, turning the trays around at the 15-minute mark.

While the puddings are baking, make the caramel sauce (refer to the Caramel Sauce recipe on page 104).

Once a skewer inserted into the centre of a pudding comes out clean, remove from the oven and let the puddings cool in the tin for 5 minutes. Gently ease the puddings out and turn them over so the pecan side is up. Place them on a cooling rack to cool completely. Drizzle caramel sauce on top and serve them warm.

RECIPE NOTES

These puddings are best served warm. The caramel sauce can be made well in advance and reheated to drizzling consistency.

These puddings freeze well in an airtight container. To reheat frozen puddings, microwave for 50 seconds to 1 minute.

Chocolate Self-Saucing Puddings

Serves 4 people

Imagine diving your spoon into the centre of a warm pudding to reveal molten, gooey chocolate sauce cascading down. This decadent treat is just right for times when you need some self-care or for that special date night with your loved one. You will not be able to resist delving into them hot out of the oven, accompanied by coconut ice-cream to finish it off.

¼ cup organic extra virgin coconut oil, melted
2 tablespoons pure maple syrup
1 tablespoon coconut sugar
1 free-range egg
1 teaspoon pure vanilla extract
½ teaspoon apple cider vinegar
⅓ cup unsweetened coconut yoghurt (vanilla flavoured)
¼ cup raw cacao powder
¼ cup nut meal (e.g. pecans, almonds, hazelnuts)
2 tablespoons teff flour
½ teaspoon baking powder
Pinch of salt

CHOCOLATE SAUCE
¾ cup boiling water
¼ cup raw cacao powder
2 tablespoons pure maple syrup
1 tablespoon coconut sugar
1 teaspoon vanilla extract
Pinch of salt

OPTIONAL TOPPING
Sprinkle coconut or maple sugar and a pinch of cinnamon over the puddings once out of the oven.

Preheat the oven to 180°C. In a mixing bowl, whisk together all of the pudding ingredients until well combined. Place two 10cm-deep ramekins on a lined baking tray, and pour the pudding mixture into the ramekins, smoothing out the tops of them.

Prepare the chocolate sauce by mixing all of the ingredients until smooth. Pour the sauce evenly over the batter in each ramekin but do not fill to the very top as this will overflow during baking and extend the cooking time.

Bake for 20-25 minutes until the puddings are bubbling and just set in the middle, but the sides are cooked. Serve immediately while they are still warm and gooey in the centre.

RECIPE NOTES

It is important to use deep ramekins to allow space for the chocolate sauce to be poured over before baking. Do not overbake the puddings or they will be fully set in the middle.

If using smaller-sized ramekins, you will need to adjust your baking times accordingly.

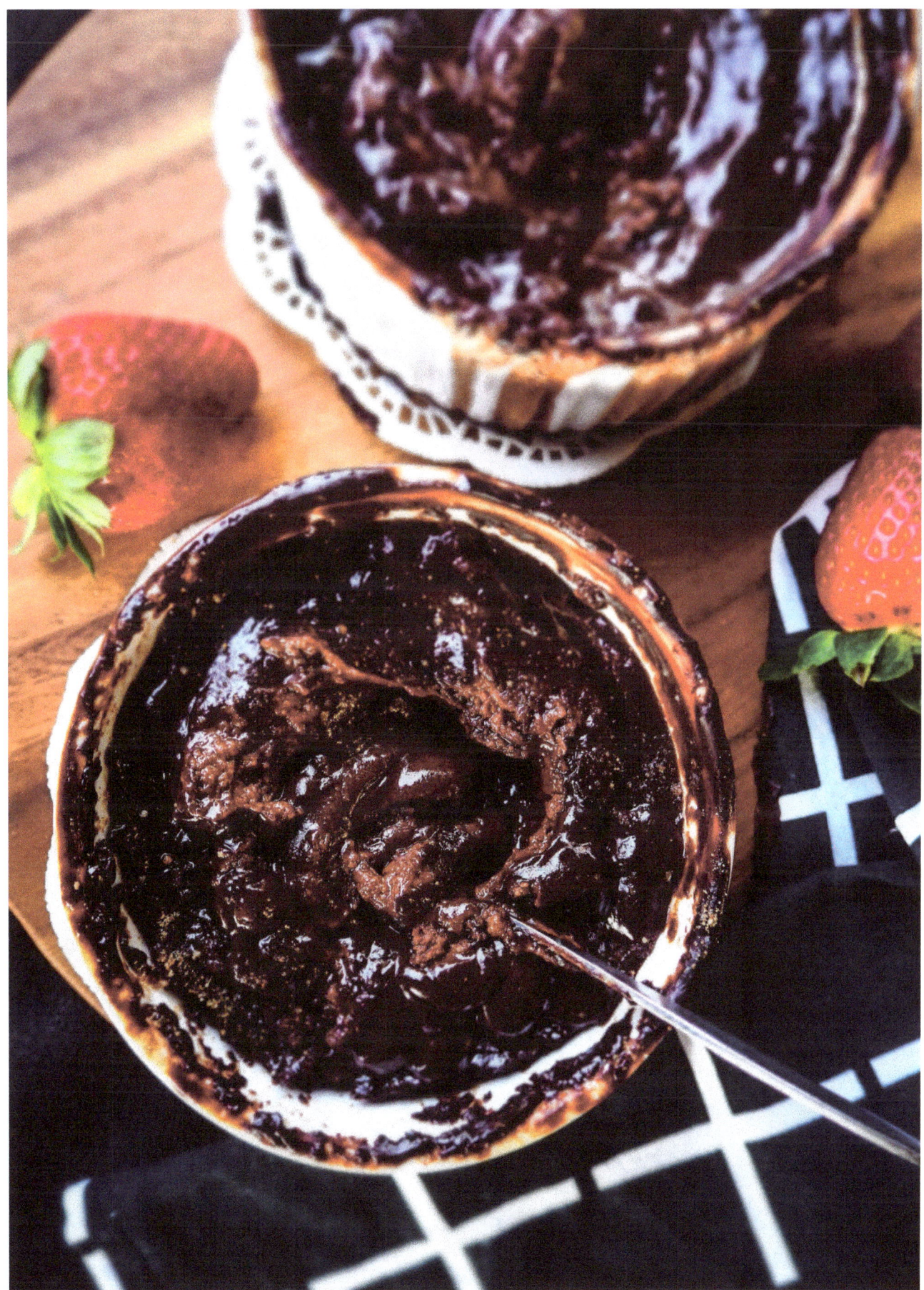

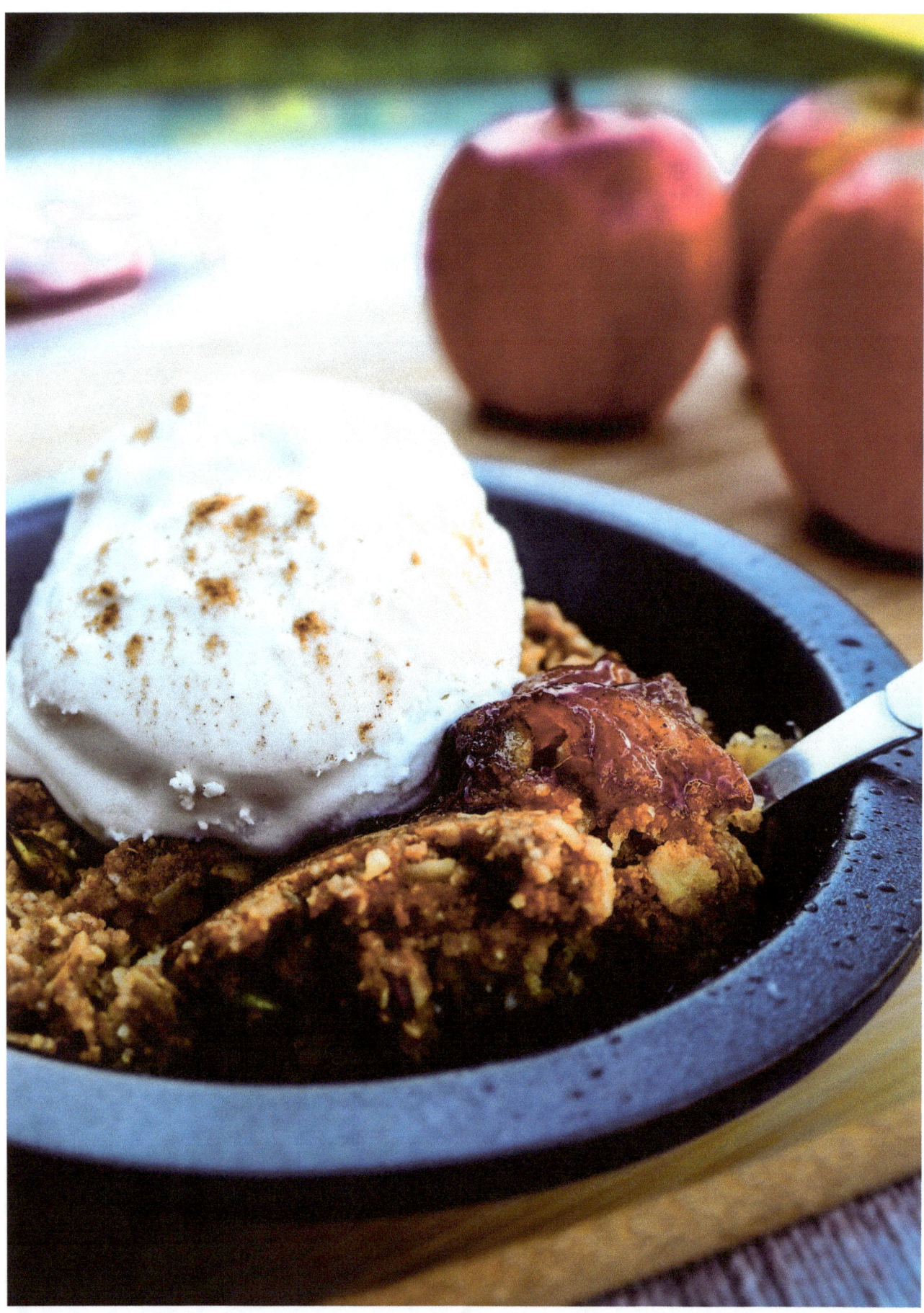

Apple Crumble

Serves 4 - 8 people

A good apple crumble has to have an equal ratio of beautifully stewed apple to a toasted, crunchy crumble. This crumble definitely has that in spades, with notes of vanilla and cinnamon throughout. Paired perfectly with some coconut ice cream or dairy-free custard, this dessert is delectably moreish!

APPLE FILLING
3 large or 4 small organic apples (I prefer to use Pink Lady), peeled and diced
½ teaspoon cinnamon powder
1 tablespoon maple syrup
1 teaspoon lemon juice
1 teaspoon vanilla extract
1 tablespoon arrowroot or tapioca starch
Pinch of salt

CRUMBLE TOPPING
1 cup almond flour
1 tablespoon coconut flour
1 tablespoon tapioca starch
½ cup heaped rolled oats
1 tablespoon coconut sugar
½ teaspoon cinnamon powder
¼ cup organic extra virgin coconut oil, melted
¼ cup maple syrup
¼ teaspoon salt

Tip: Add pepitas, sunflower seeds or chopped nuts for crunch.

Preheat the oven to 190°c and grease 4-6 medium-sized ramekins or 8 small ramekins or mini pie tins with organic extra virgin coconut oil.

Peel apples and dice into small cubes or slice thinly if preferred. In a mixing bowl, mix together all apple filling ingredients. Set aside.

In a separate bowl, mix together the crumble ingredients until small clumps form.

Fill each ramekin or mini pie tin with apple filling and top each one with the crumble.

Bake at 190°c for 30-40 minutes until the crumble is golden brown.

RECIPE NOTES

Makes filling for approximately 4-6 medium-sized ramekins or 8 small ramekins.

If having leftovers:
From the fridge — Reheat at 150°c for 20 minutes.
From the freezer — Reheat at 150°c for 30 minutes.

You can freeze the pre-mixed unbaked crumble in an airtight container or ziplock bag for use when needed. You can also freeze the baked apple crumble by wrapping the ramekins or mini pie tins with cling wrap, followed by a layer of foil to keep it airtight.

BREADS, PASTRY & CEREALS

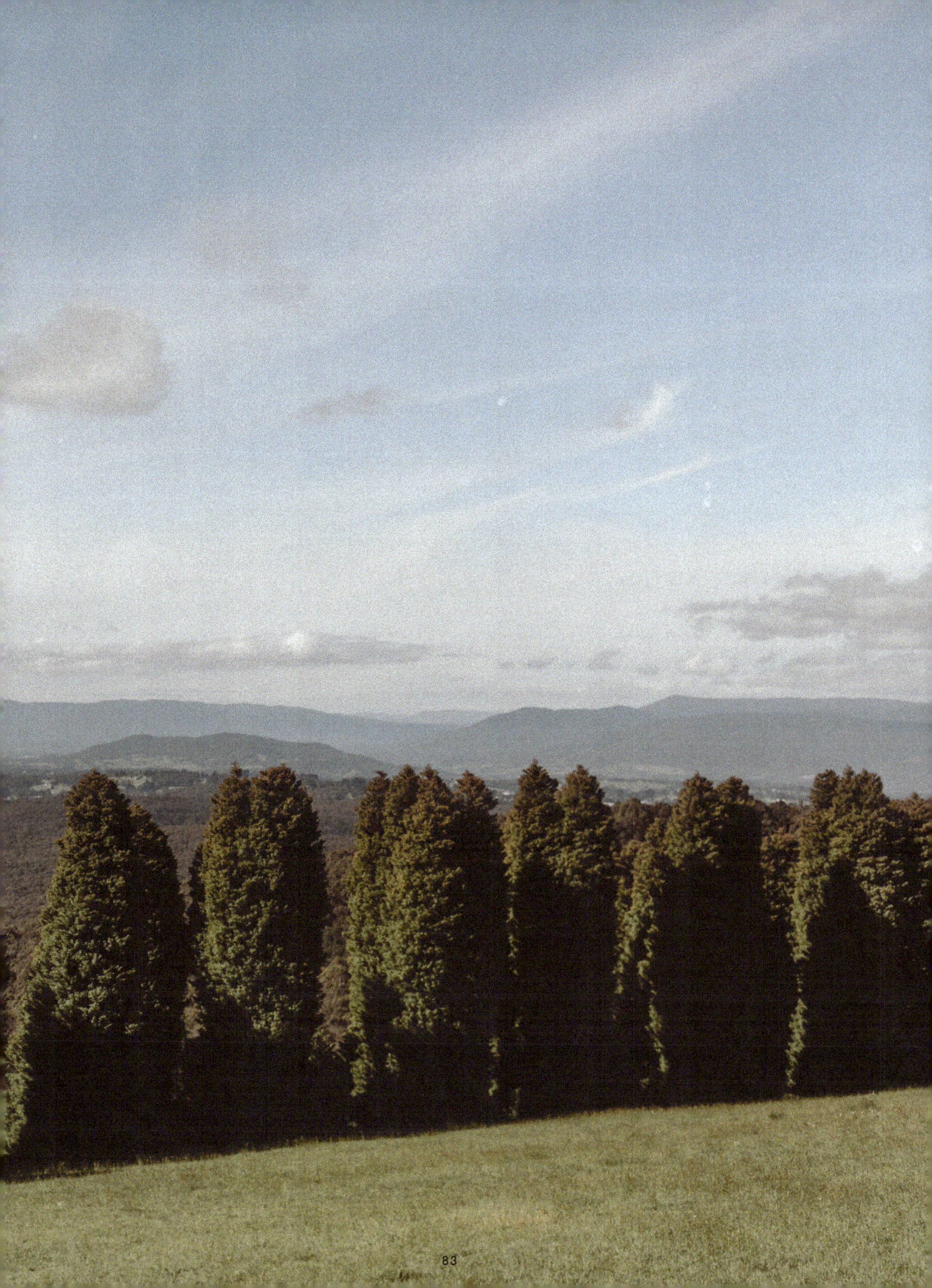

Gluten-Free Flour Blend — Option 1

Makes 500 g

The general rule of thumb in any gluten-free flour blend is that it needs to comprise a 40% wholegrain flour to 60% starch ratio. This will ensure the best texture and result in your baked goods. It is also important to use all organic and GMO (Genetically Modified Organism)-free flours and starches as much as possible. The below flour options are suitable for use on their own or in combination with other flours such as almond flour, quinoa flour, oat flour, green banana flour, tiger nut flour or cassava flour.

MIX TOGETHER:

WHOLE GRAIN FLOUR
1 ¾ cups brown rice flour

STARCHES
½ cup potato starch
¼ cup tapioca starch or arrowroot starch

This is a good flour blend to use when you need to batter fish or dust a board before kneading dough. It is also good for when a recipe calls for added flour to thicken and bind, such as in fritters or frittata. Store the flour in an airtight container in a cool environment away from direct sunlight.

Gluten-Free Flour Blend — Option 2

Makes 1 kg

MIX TOGETHER:

WHOLE GRAIN FLOURS
1 cup millet flour (can substitute with 1 cup brown rice flour or 1 ¼ cups oat flour)
1 cup sorghum flour
Heaped ¾ cup teff flour

STARCHES
1 cup & 2 tablespoons potato starch
1 ½ cups glutinous rice flour
1 ½ cups arrowroot starch or tapioca starch

This flour blend is ideal to use for when you just want a quick substitute for wheat flour in a recipe and require a good amount of it, too. It is also nutrient-packed and is perfect to use for biscuits, scones, cakes and the like. Store the flour in an airtight container or large ziplock bag in the fridge to maintain freshness.

Slice and Tart Base — Option 1

Makes 1 standard-sized tart shell or slice base

This pastry dough is ideal for creating textured, oat-like bases with substance and can be used to make slices and tarts. It provides a similar feel to a cheesecake base made of crushed digestive biscuits, with a good crunch.

1 cup oat flour
½ cup almond flour
½ cup teff flour
¼ cup arrowroot starch
⅓ cup organic extra virgin coconut oil (cold, scoopable)
¼ cup pure maple syrup
½ teaspoon salt
½ teaspoon pure vanilla extract
1 teaspoon apple cider vinegar

Preheat the oven to 200°c. In a mixing bowl, combine all the ingredients together to form a sticky but pliable dough. Add water if the dough feels too dry.

Using whichever-sized baking tin that the recipe calls for, press and mould the dough into the tin and use a fork to create holes in the bottom to prevent it from puffing up during baking. Blind bake the pastry for 20 minutes.

Once the pastry is out of the oven, reduce the oven temperature to 175°c or as the recipe directs. If the pastry has shrunk a little on the sides, just gently press the sides in with your fingers to raise it again. Make the filling and pour over the cooled pastry shell or base.

Return to the oven to bake for another 30-40 minutes or as indicated in the recipe. Let it cool before serving.

Slice and Tart Base — Option 2

Makes 1 standard-sized tart shell or slice base

This pastry dough is very similar to a shortcrust pastry and is perfect to use as a tart shell for savoury and sweet fillings. Depending on the recipe it is used for, the results of the pastry can be light and flaky or sturdier with a wonderful crumb.

½ cup organic extra virgin coconut oil (cold, scoopable) or 100 g vegan butter (cold, cubed)
½ teaspoon salt
1 free-range egg
2 tablespoons golden flaxseed meal
1 tablespoon ice-cold water
2 tablespoons maple sugar or coconut sugar
¼ cup almond flour or quinoa flour
¼ cup Gluten-Free Flour Blend — Option 1
¾ cup sorghum flour
1 teaspoon apple cider vinegar
1 teaspoon pure vanilla extract (if encasing a sweet filling)

Preheat the oven to 190°c. In a food processor, combine all the ingredients together and blitz until it starts to come together. Turn out the dough onto a board and bring it all together until a smooth ball of dough is formed. Cling wrap and refrigerate for 1 hour to allow the dough to rest.

Once the dough has rested, take it out and place it on a generously-floured board. Dust the dough lightly with some gluten-free flour, then roll it out to the desired thickness according to the recipe.

Alternatively, if the dough is a little on the soft side once out of the fridge, dust the dough with some gluten-free flour and give it a little knead. Using whichever-sized baking tin that the recipe calls for, place the dough into the tart tin and press and shape it into the mould nicely, making sure the desired thickness is even on all sides and the bottom, appropriate to the recipe. This process is slightly more labour-intensive, but the results will be the same. Use a fork to create holes in the bottom to prevent it from puffing up during baking. Blind bake the pastry for 15 minutes.

Once the pastry is out of the oven, reduce the oven temperature to 175°c or as the recipe directs. Make the filling and pour over the cooled pastry shell or base. Return to the oven to bake for another 45 minutes or as indicated in the recipe. Let it cool before serving.

Slice and Tart Base — Option 3

Makes 1 standard-sized tart shell or slice base

This fabulous shortbread pastry is deliciously rich and crumbly, with a cookie-like texture that melts in your mouth. Even with its delicate form, it is an ideal foundation for sweet tarts and slices.

1 cup almond flour
½ cup sorghum flour
¼ cup tapioca starch
¼ cup brown rice flour
2 tablespoons coconut flour
⅓ cup organic extra virgin coconut oil, melted
⅓ cup pure maple syrup
1 teaspoon pure vanilla extract
½ teaspoon pure almond extract
¼ teaspoon salt

Preheat the oven to 180°c. In a mixing bowl, combine all the ingredients together to form a sticky but pliable dough.

Using whichever-sized baking tin the recipe calls for, press and mould the dough into the tin and use a fork to create holes in the base to prevent it from puffing up during baking. Bake the pastry for 20-25 minutes until golden brown.

Once the pastry is out of the oven, let it cool while making the filling. Pour the filling over the cooled pastry shell or base. Follow the remaining instructions as per the recipe.

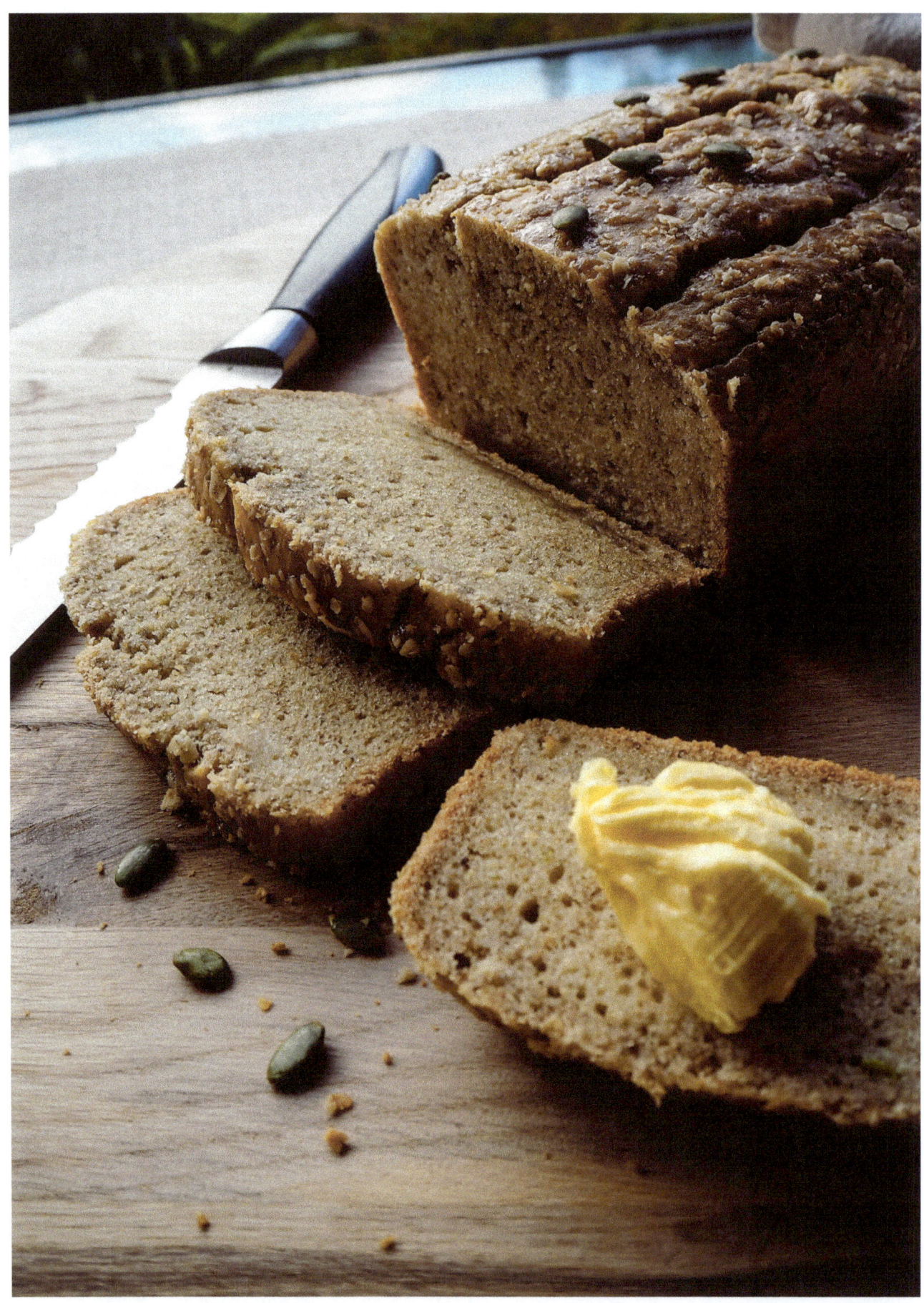

Gluten & Yeast-Free Sandwich Bread Loaf

Makes 1 loaf

It has taken many experimental bread-making days to achieve the ultimate sandwich bread that is both gluten-free and yeast-free, yet tastes and feels like an artisanal rye loaf. Marked by its beautiful springy texture and crust, with its soft and light crumbs; it even has the little air pockets throughout the inside that resembles its gluten counterparts. This bread is delightful - untoasted or as a toastie.

1 cup unsweetened plain coconut yoghurt
½ cup unsweetened almond milk
4 tablespoons olive oil
2 tablespoons pure maple syrup
½ teaspoon salt
1 cup tapioca starch
½ cup arrowroot starch
¼ cup millet or sorghum flour
¼ cup oat flour
½ cup brown rice flour
⅓ cup potato starch
2 tablespoons glutinous rice flour
2 ¼ teaspoons baking powder
½ teaspoon baking soda
2 teaspoons apple cider vinegar
3 free-range egg whites
2 tablespoons golden flaxseed meal
2 tablespoons milled sunflower and/or pepita seeds

Preheat the oven to 190°C and grease a 24 cm x 14 cm bread loaf tin.

In a mixing bowl, whisk together coconut yoghurt, almond milk, olive oil, maple syrup and salt together until well combined. Add in the gluten-free flours and mix until a dough forms.

In a separate bowl, beat the egg whites with the apple cider vinegar using an electric or handheld mixer and whisk until stiff peaks form. Fold in the egg white mix, baking powder, baking soda, flaxseed meal and milled seeds into the dough until just combined. This will form a slightly wet dough.

Pour the wet dough into the greased bread loaf tin and smooth the top to avoid large cracks. If preferred, sprinkle some rolled oats on top.

Bake for 1 hour and 15 minutes, or until a skewer inserted into the centre of the bread comes out clean.

Once removed from the oven, allow the bread to cool in the tin for 5 minutes before turning it out onto a wire rack to cool completely. This will avoid condensation build-up and ensure the bottom crust does not become soggy. Allow to cool completely before slicing (approximately 4 hours).

RECIPE NOTES

It is important to allow the bread to cool down completely before slicing, as slicing it prematurely will result in a gummy texture due to less resting time.

To preserve the freshness of the bread, slice all the way through and place bread slices in an airtight container and refrigerate. It also freezes well.

Pita Flatbread Wraps

Makes 5 average-sized wraps

These pita flatbread wraps remind me of roti, commonly prepared in Indian and Thai cuisines. They are crispy around the edges and chewy with the perfect textural bend to use as taco shells or as your favourite lunch wrap. A bonus is the use of the green banana flour, which provides a superb source of prebiotics to help feed the good bacteria in your gut. Be creative with the fillings and get wrapping!

¼ cup millet flour or brown rice flour
¼ cup green banana flour
½ cup tapioca or arrowroot starch
1 cup unsweetened almond milk or coconut milk
¼ teaspoon salt
2 teaspoons coconut flour
Optional add-in: fresh or dried chives

Combine all ingredients together in a mixing bowl until a smooth batter is formed.

In a non-stick frying pan, drizzle about 2 teaspoons of olive oil and garlic-infused olive oil over medium heat. Do not add too much oil as this makes the flatbread oily and not as light in texture.

Using a soup ladle, spoon a ladle-sized batter into the frying pan, spreading it out into a rough circle. Allow it to cook for 1-2 minutes, before flipping it over to cook on the other side. Flip the wrap around 4-6 times until it is golden and crispy. Remove and lay the wrap on a tray and place in a warmed oven while cooking the other wraps, so it stays crispy and warm.

Top your wraps with your choice of savoury condiments and fillings.

RECIPE NOTES

These wraps are best eaten fresh on the day they are made.

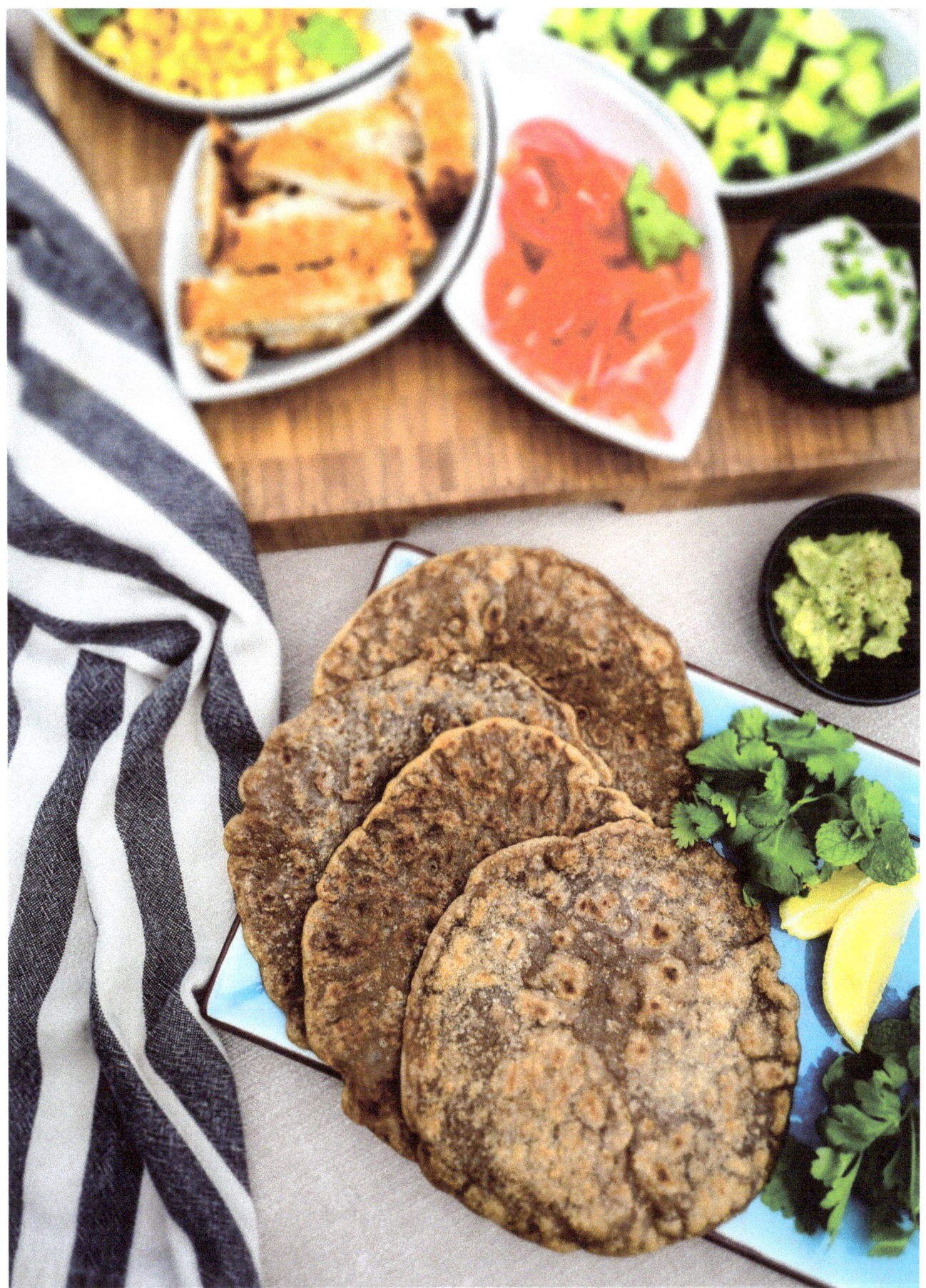

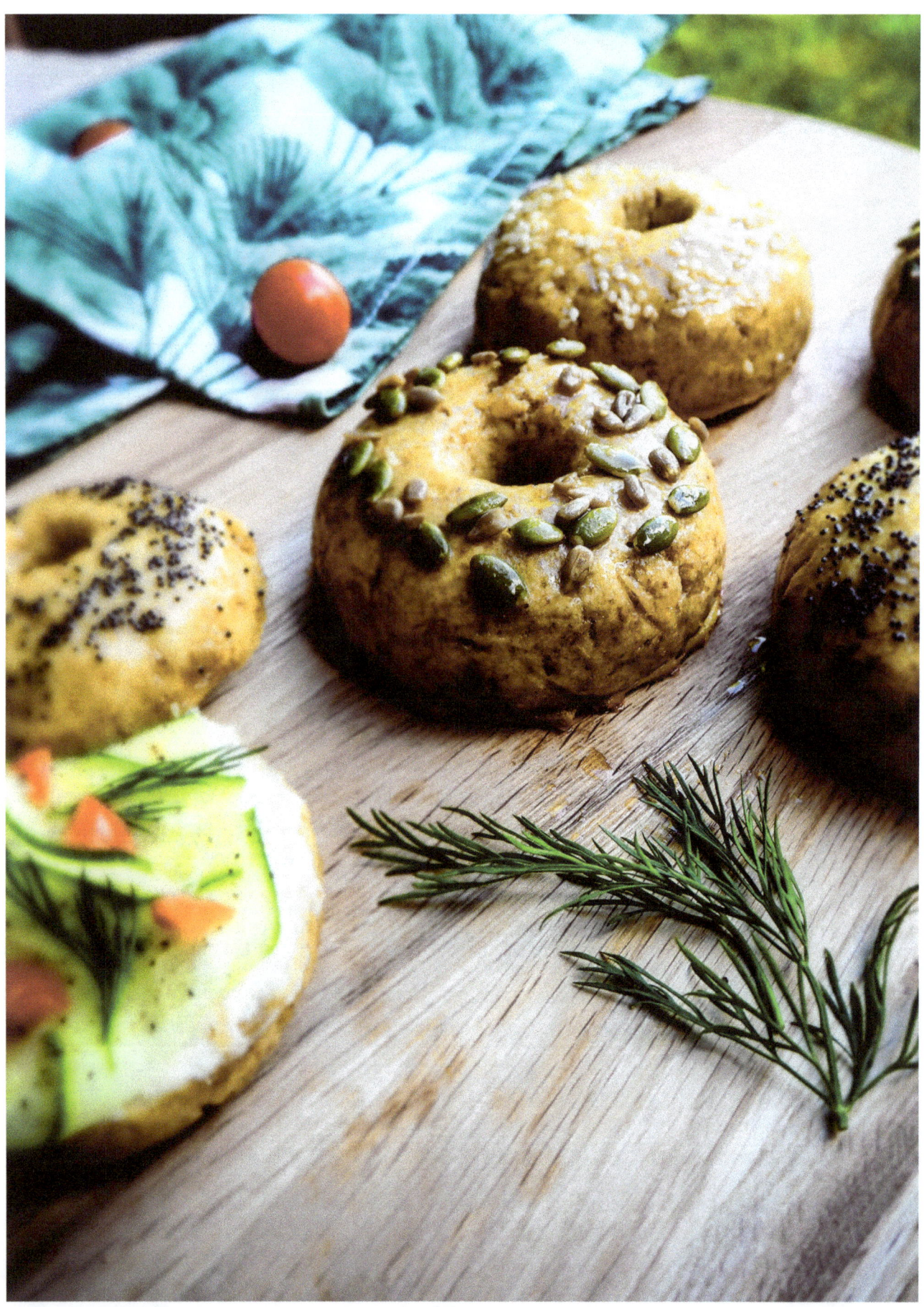

Gluten-Free Bagels

Makes 6 bagels

These bagels have just the right density but are surprisingly light with a good crumb on the inside. Whether they are eaten straight out of the oven and on their own, used as an accompaniment to a soup, or toasted and devoured with your sweet or savoury topping of choice; these bagels are sure to become an all-year favourite.

½ cup cassava flour
½ cup arrowroot starch
½ cup almond flour (not meal)
¼ cup oat flour
¼ cup quinoa flour
2 tablespoons potato starch
4 tablespoons glutinous rice flour
1 tablespoon golden flaxseed meal
2 tablespoons hot water
4 free-range eggs
¼ cup organic extra virgin coconut oil or olive oil
2 tablespoons pure maple syrup
1 teaspoon baking powder
½ teaspoon salt
1-2 tablespoons water (if the dough is too dry)

TOPPING
Sesame seeds, poppy seeds, pepitas, sunflower seeds

EGG WASH
1 free-range egg
1 tablespoon almond milk

Preheat the oven to 175°c and line a baking tray. Fill a large saucepan halfway with water and bring to a boil. Lower the fire but keep water boiling.

Mix the tablespoon of flaxseed meal with 2 tablespoons of hot water and let sit for 5-10 minutes to thicken to a gel consistency.

Combine all ingredients in a bowl, including the flaxseed gel, and knead until smooth. The dough will be sticky, so let it rest for about 5 minutes until workable.

Using a spatula, separate the dough into 6 equal parts. To ensure the dough does not stick too much on your hands, lightly oil your hands before rolling each segment of dough into a ball. Working on a clean food board, flatten the ball of dough slightly and mould it into the shape of a doughnut. Use a chopstick or your index finger to make a hole in the middle, making sure the bagel is smooth all over, with no rough edges.

Using a large slotted spoon, lower one bagel at a time into the boiling water and cook for 1 minute until it rises to the top. Once the bagel floats, flip it over and cook the other side for 1 minute.

As each bagel is boiled, place them on the lined baking tray, 3 cm apart, 2 per row. Brush with the egg wash and sprinkle with desired toppings. Bake at 175°c for 25 minutes until lightly golden brown.

Remove the bagels to cool on a wire rack for 20 minutes before cutting and eating.

RECIPE NOTES

The dough should be sticky like cookie dough, not like bread dough. However, once mixed, let it rest for about 5 minutes to firm up before rolling into 6 balls to form the doughnut shape.

Bagels will toast well. Slice in half and freeze in a zip-lock bag or an airtight container to prevent them from drying out.

Scones

Makes 7-9 scones

These any-season teatime delights are deliciously moist with a good crumb and a hint of lemon. They are super easy to make and pair wonderfully with your favourite condiments of dairy-free butter, jam or coconut cream.

1 ½ cups Gluten-Free Flour Blend — Option 2
¼ cup almond flour or tiger nut flour
¼ cup oat flour
1 ½ teaspoons baking powder
¼ teaspoon salt
1 tablespoon golden flaxseed meal
2 tablespoons pure maple syrup or coconut sugar
1 teaspoon pure vanilla extract
½ teaspoon apple cider vinegar
The rind of 1 lemon
125 g cold vegan butter, cubed
½ cup unsweetened coconut yoghurt (vanilla flavour is optional)
4 tablespoons unsweetened almond milk

OPTIONAL ADD-INS
¼ cup dried cranberries, sultanas or blueberries (sulphite-free)

EGG WASH
1 egg
1 teaspoon almond milk

Preheat the oven to 200°c and line a baking tin. In a mixing bowl, mix flour, baking powder, salt and lemon rind together until combined. Using your fingers, rub in vegan butter into the flour mixture until it resembles a crumb-like consistency. You can use a food processor to blitz it altogether if you prefer.

Make a well in the centre of the dry crumb mixture and add in the coconut yoghurt, almond milk, apple cider vinegar, vanilla extract and maple syrup or coconut sugar.

Using your hands or a wooden spoon, stir until just combined. The dough will be quite wet. Pour the dough onto a floured surface (I use brown rice flour to dust generously) and knead the dough gently until it is just coming together. Be sure not to over-knead the dough.

Flatten the dough to about 3 cm thick. Using a 6.5 cm diameter scone or cookie cutter, dip the cutting edge in flour before cutting rounds in the dough until all the dough is used up. This will ensure the dough does not stick to the cutter when trying to release it on the baking tray. You will need to re-group the dough and flatten it to make more rounds as you go, dusting the board every so often to ensure it does not stick.

Place each round of dough onto the lined baking tray, with each portion just touching each other. This will help them to rise better. Brush each scone with egg wash and bake at 200°c for 22 minutes until lightly golden brown.

Once the scones are out of the oven, cover them with a tea towel to prevent them from drying out. Serve with your favourite condiments or enjoy them on their own.

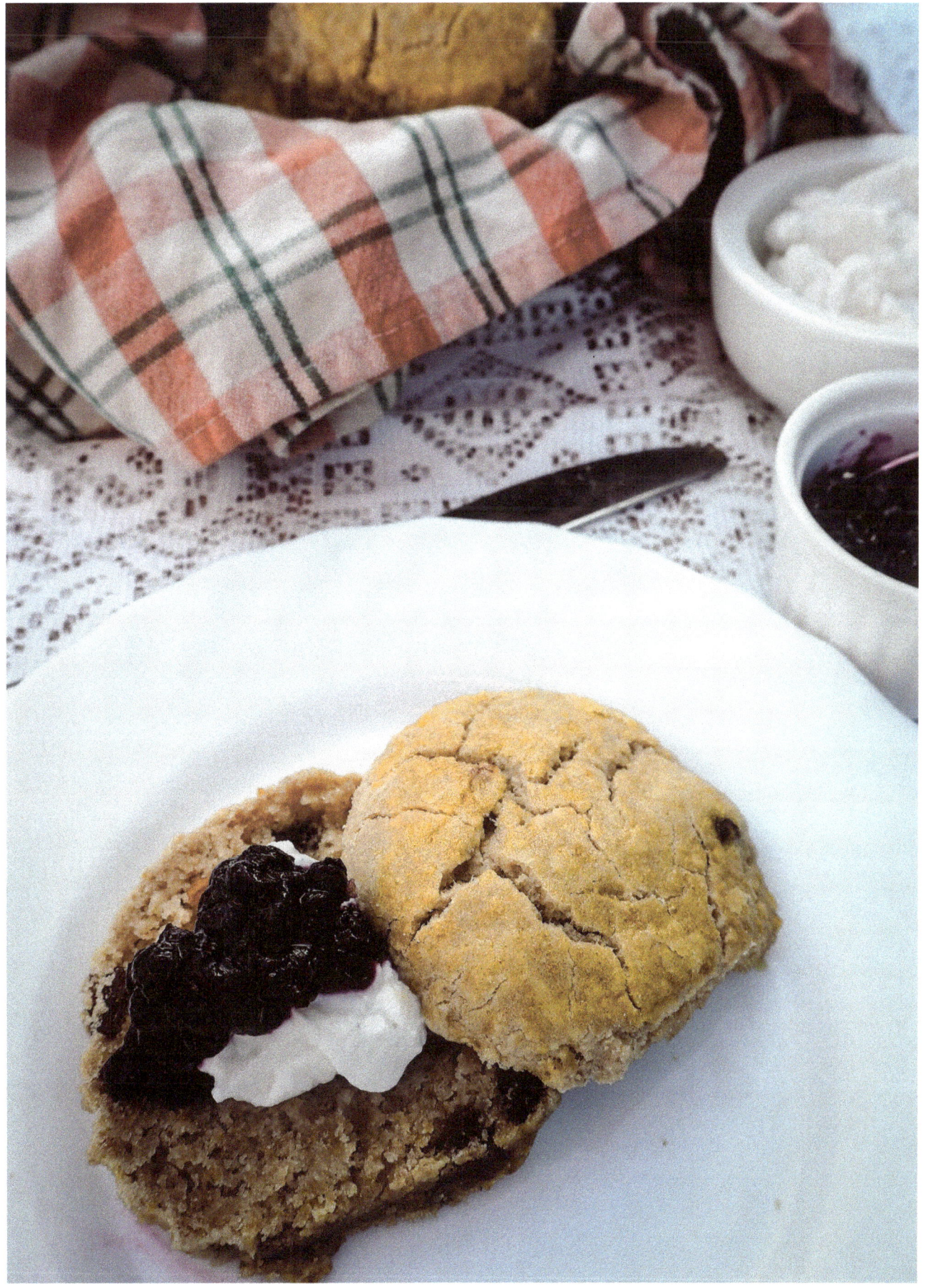

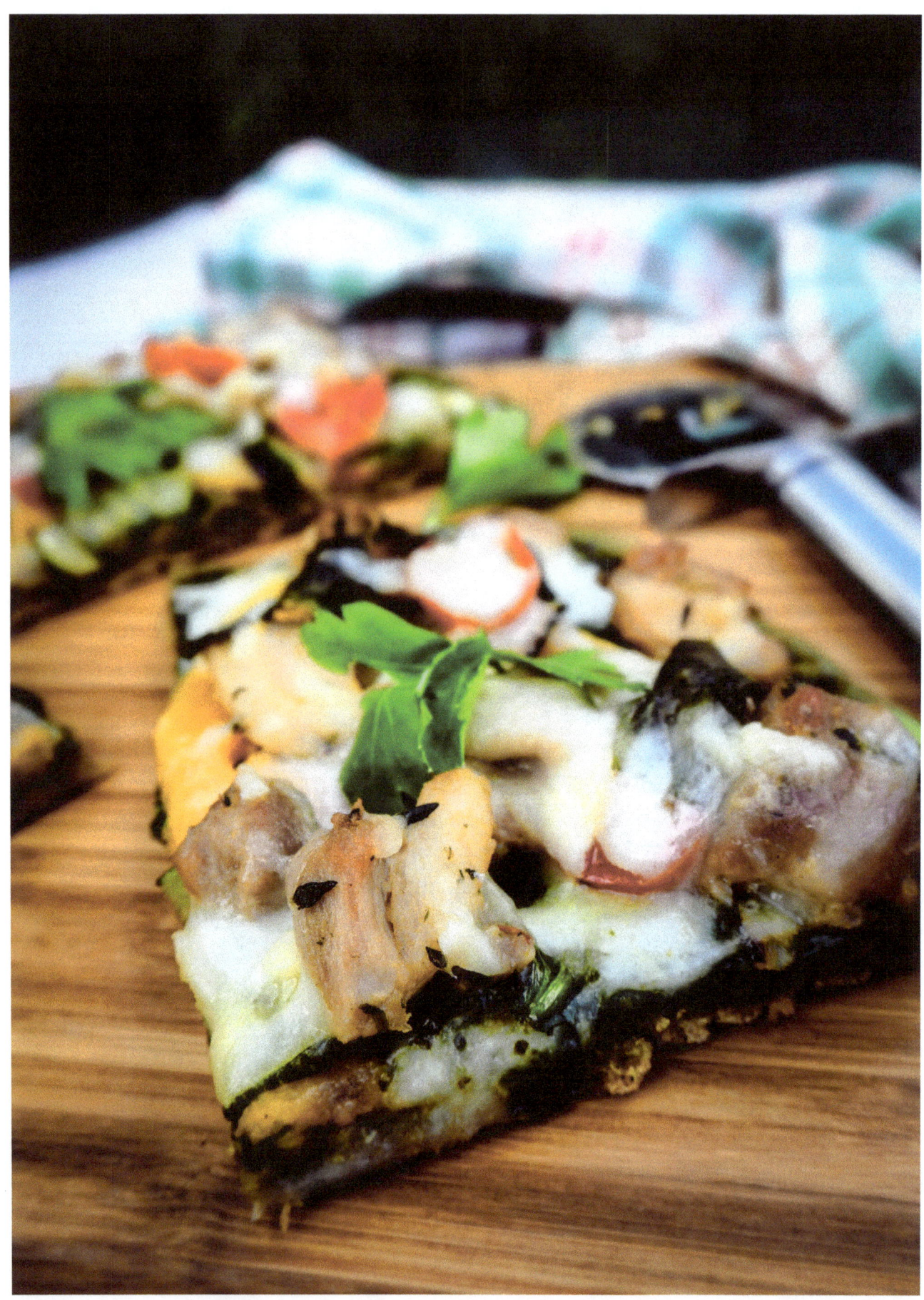

Gluten-Free Pizza Bases

Makes 1 large and 2 medium-sized pizza bases

I don't know about you, but I like my pizza bases to be thin and crispy, yet bready with a good stretch and bend to be able to withstand any amount of toppings you desire. These pizza bases fit the bill, plus they are incredibly healthy and tasty. Why not make them on your next pizza night and get creative with your topping options!

¼ cup teff flour
½ cup oat flour
¼ cup quinoa flour
¼ cup cassava flour
¼ cup sorghum flour
½ cup brown rice flour
¼ cup potato starch
½ cup tapioca starch or arrowroot starch
2 tablespoons glutinous rice flour
¾ teaspoon sea salt
1 free-range egg
2 tablespoons golden flaxseed meal
4 tablespoons hot water
2 teaspoons pure maple syrup
1 cup unsweetened almond milk
1 cup water
2 tablespoons olive oil

Preheat the oven to 180°c and line 3 trays with baking paper. In a bowl, mix the golden flaxseed meal with the boiling water and let sit for 5 minutes.

In a large mixing bowl, whisk together all the flours and salt until well blended. Whisk the flaxseed gel, egg, maple syrup, almond milk, water and olive oil together thoroughly and pour into the dry ingredients. Continue whisking until a smooth batter is formed. It should share the same consistency as pancake batter.

Drizzle and smear a little olive oil onto the baking papers on each tray and pour the batter evenly onto each tray. Using a spatula, ensure the batter is 3-5 mm thick and spread out in a rectangular shape. This should make 4 medium-sized pizzas or 1 large and 2 medium pizzas. Place the pizza bases in the oven to blind bake for 10 minutes.

Remove and place desired toppings then return to the oven to bake for a further 20- 25 minutes. Once out of the oven, slice and serve immediately.

RECIPE NOTES

These pizza bases freeze well. To reheat from frozen, heat up for 25 minutes at 160°c.

Suggested toppings:

- Chicken pesto, pumpkin, zucchini, tuscan kale and dairy-free or low-lactose cheese.
- Garlic olive oil with parsley, chives, fresh basil and dairy-free or low-lactose cheese.
- Lamb, spaghetti squash, tuscan kale and fresh herbs, drizzled with coconut yoghurt.

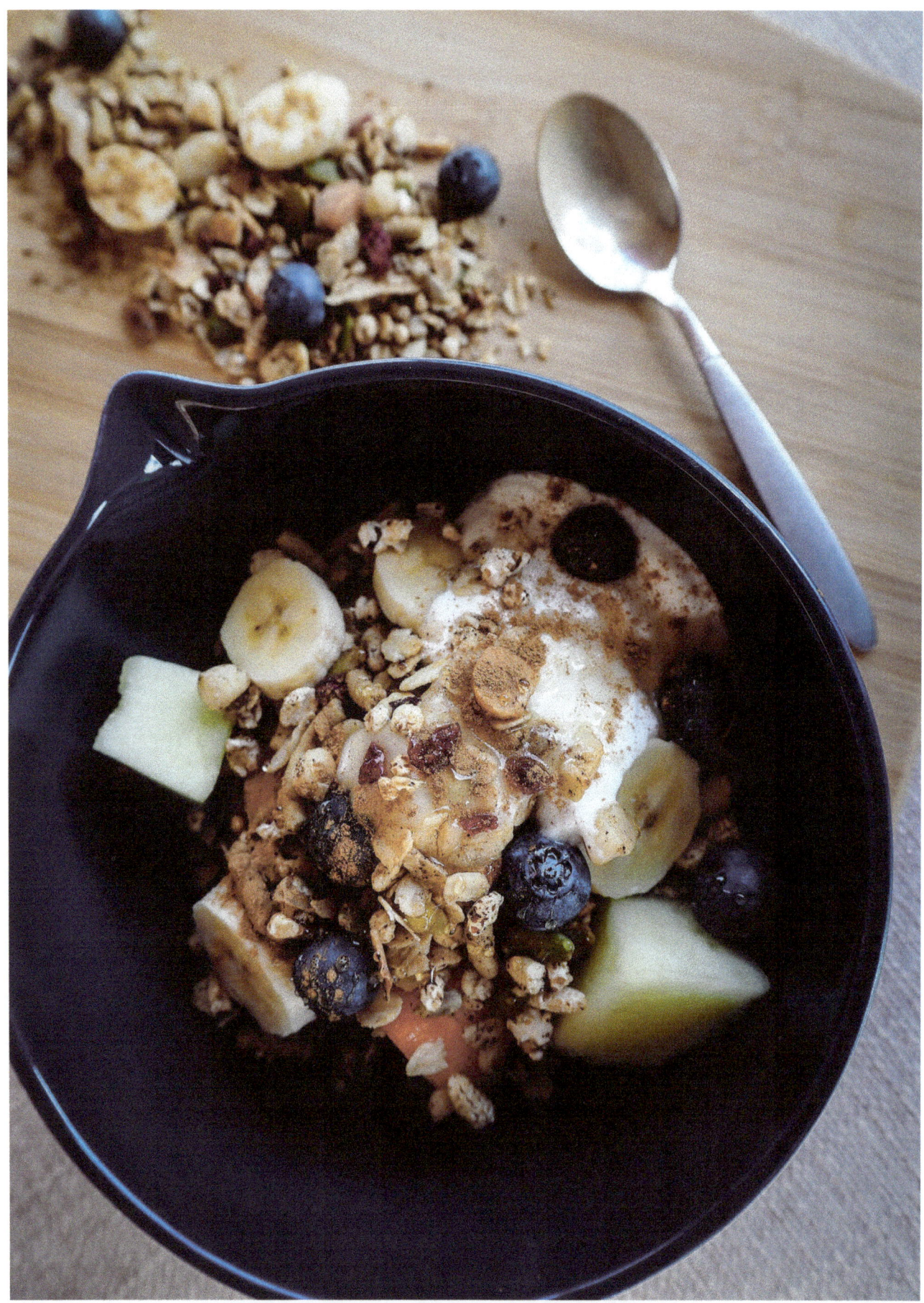

Muesli

Makes 5.5 litres

Muesli is a great way to start the day, for a healthy mid-morning or afternoon snack. It is great on its own with milk or yoghurt, or mix it up by serving it with some fresh fruit. If you like it a tad sweeter, drizzle a little extra maple syrup on top before serving. As it is packed with heart-healthy oats, nuts, seeds and mixed ancient grains, a little goes a long way to keep you satisfied and full of energy. This is also a brilliant way to get some much-needed fibre and protein into your diet. Give me homemade muesli any day of the week.

½ cup heaped organic extra virgin coconut oil, melted
⅔ heaped cup pure maple syrup
2 teaspoons pure vanilla extract
½ teaspoon salt
4 cups organic rolled oats
1 cup organic puffed millet
1 cup organic puffed quinoa
3 cups mixed puffed cereal
½ cup rice bran cereal
3 cups chopped mixed nuts and seeds
½ cup dried cranberries, chopped (or any other dried fruit of choice)
2 tablespoons hemp flour
4 tablespoons golden flaxseed meal
1 teaspoon cinnamon powder

Preheat the oven to 165°c and line 3 trays with baking paper. In a large mixing bowl, combine all the dry ingredients together (except for the dried cranberries).

Heat the coconut oil, maple syrup, salt and vanilla extract over medium heat for 2-3 minutes, until bubbling and frothy. Remove from heat and pour the maple mixture over the dry ingredients. Stir thoroughly to ensure even coating of syrup throughout the muesli.

Spread the muesli out evenly across the 3 lined trays. Bake at 165°c for 15 minutes. Remove from the oven and give the muesli a toss with a spatula to ensure even toasting and to avoid burning. Return to the oven and bake for a further 15 minutes.

Remove trays from the oven. The muesli should be nicely toasted and will crispen up as it cools down. Once the muesli has cooled down slightly, stir in the dried cranberries. Allow to cool completely before transferring into 2 airtight containers.

RECIPE NOTES

For the mixed nuts and seeds, I use pecans, macadamias, almonds, hazelnuts, brazil nuts, sunflower seeds and pepita seeds.

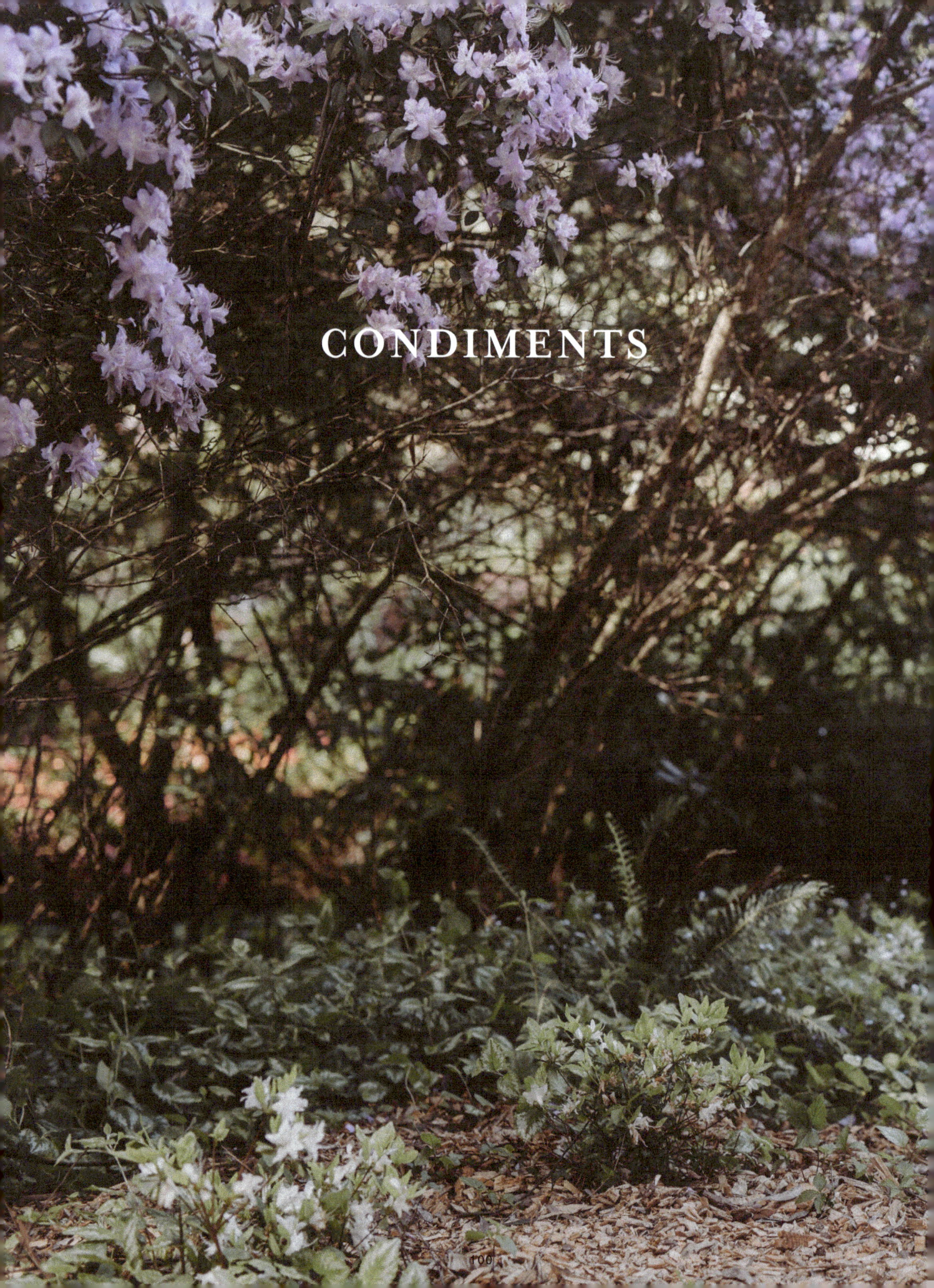
CONDIMENTS

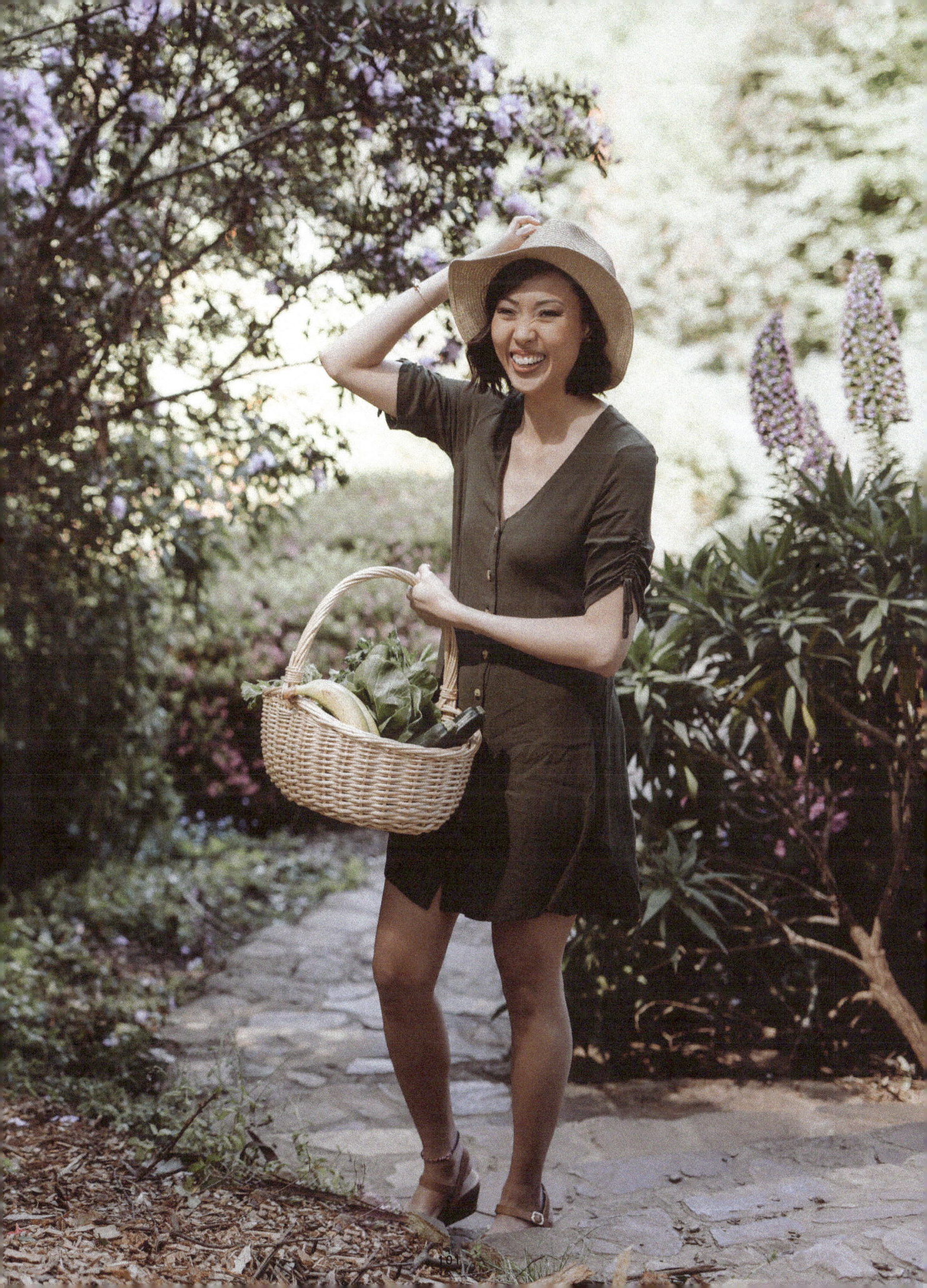

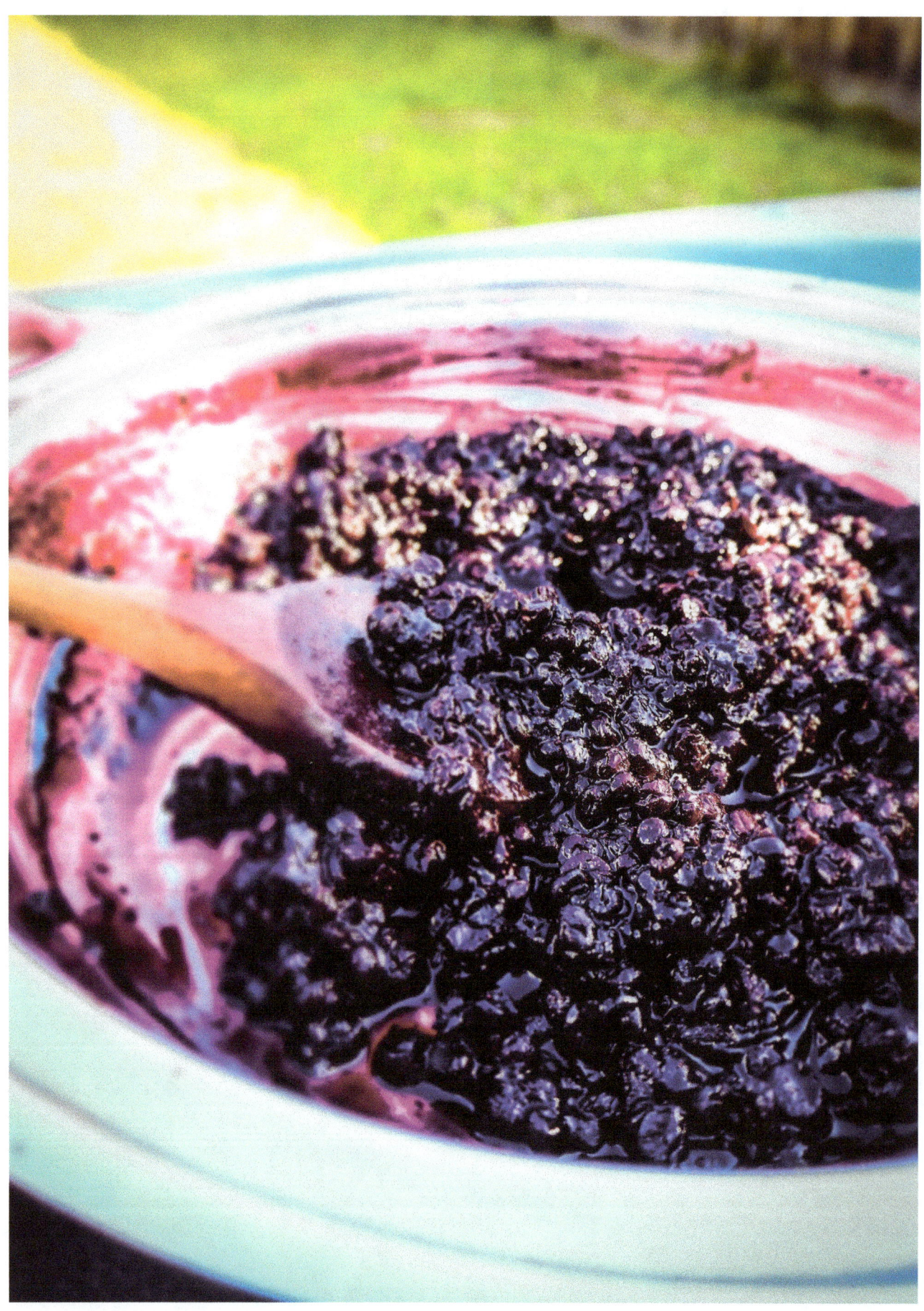

Blueberry Jam

Makes 2 average-sized jars

My love for blueberries began when I discovered they are a safe low-histamine fruit I can eat plenty of. Best of all, they are packed with antioxidants which have many amazing health benefits! This blueberry jam has the right balance of sweetness and acidity, is refined sugar-free and without artificial preservatives or thickening agents; reduced naturally and slowly to produce a thick, glossy texture and wonderful depth of flavour. It is so versatile and can go in just about anything. It is a perfect topping on pancakes, toast, brownies, scones or crackers, and pairs very well with dark chocolate.

4 ¼ heaped cups organic blueberries, fresh or frozen
⅔ cups pure maple syrup
Juice of ½ lemon or 1 tablespoon apple cider vinegar
1 teaspoon pure vanilla extract (optional)
The rind of 1 lemon
Pinch of salt

Add all ingredients into a stainless steel frying pan. Place on the stove and heat on medium heat.

As the blueberries begin to heat, mash them gently to break them down (I use a potato masher as I find it does the job well). Once the jam starts to simmer, turn to low heat and cook for approximately 45 minutes until it thickens, stirring frequently. You should be able to create a line on the back of a wooden spoon without the jam coming together quickly.

Remove from the stove top and let the jam cool for about 30 minutes before pouring it into jars. Allow them to cool further before placing them in the fridge.

RECIPE NOTES

If histamines are not an issue, you can mix with strawberries or mixed berries.

If using frozen berries, it will take longer to cook as there is more liquid, but ensure berries are sufficiently defrosted before cooking.

The jam should last 3-4 weeks in the fridge.

Caramel Sauce

Makes 1 average-sized jar

I am always blown away by how decadently rich this caramel sauce is, with the perfect combination of sweet and salty. The addition of the tahini, almond butter or sunflower seed butter provides an extra depth of flavour. This caramel sauce mirrors a dulce de leche, and is perfect to use in tarts and slices, and drizzled on puddings or pancakes. Best of all, it is so easy to make!

¼ cup coconut sugar
¼ cup pure maple syrup
2 tablespoons water
2 tablespoons tahini or almond butter or sunflower seed butter
2 tablespoons organic extra virgin coconut oil, solid
¼ teaspoons salt
½ teaspoon pure vanilla extract

In a saucepan, heat coconut sugar, maple syrup and water over medium heat until sugar dissolves completely and starts to bubble. Allow to simmer for 2-3 minutes without stirring.

Remove from heat and add in tahini or almond butter or sunflower seed butter, salt, coconut oil and vanilla extract. Using a whisk, stir to combine.

Use immediately or store caramel in a glass bottle in the fridge. It will thicken up nicely as it cools down.

RECIPE NOTES

It can keep for up to a month, refrigerated.

To soften the caramel sauce to a drizzle consistency, microwave for 15-20 seconds.

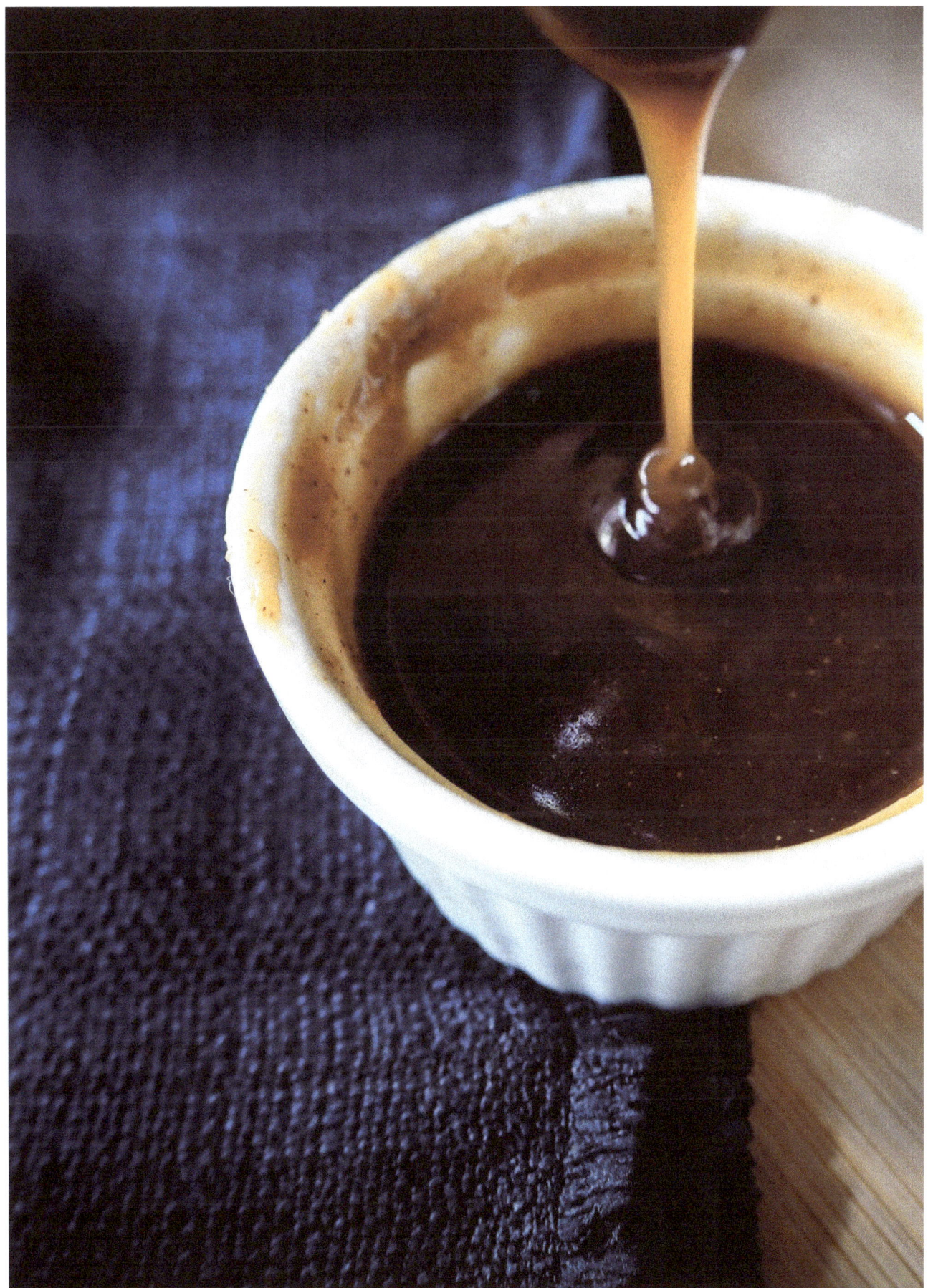

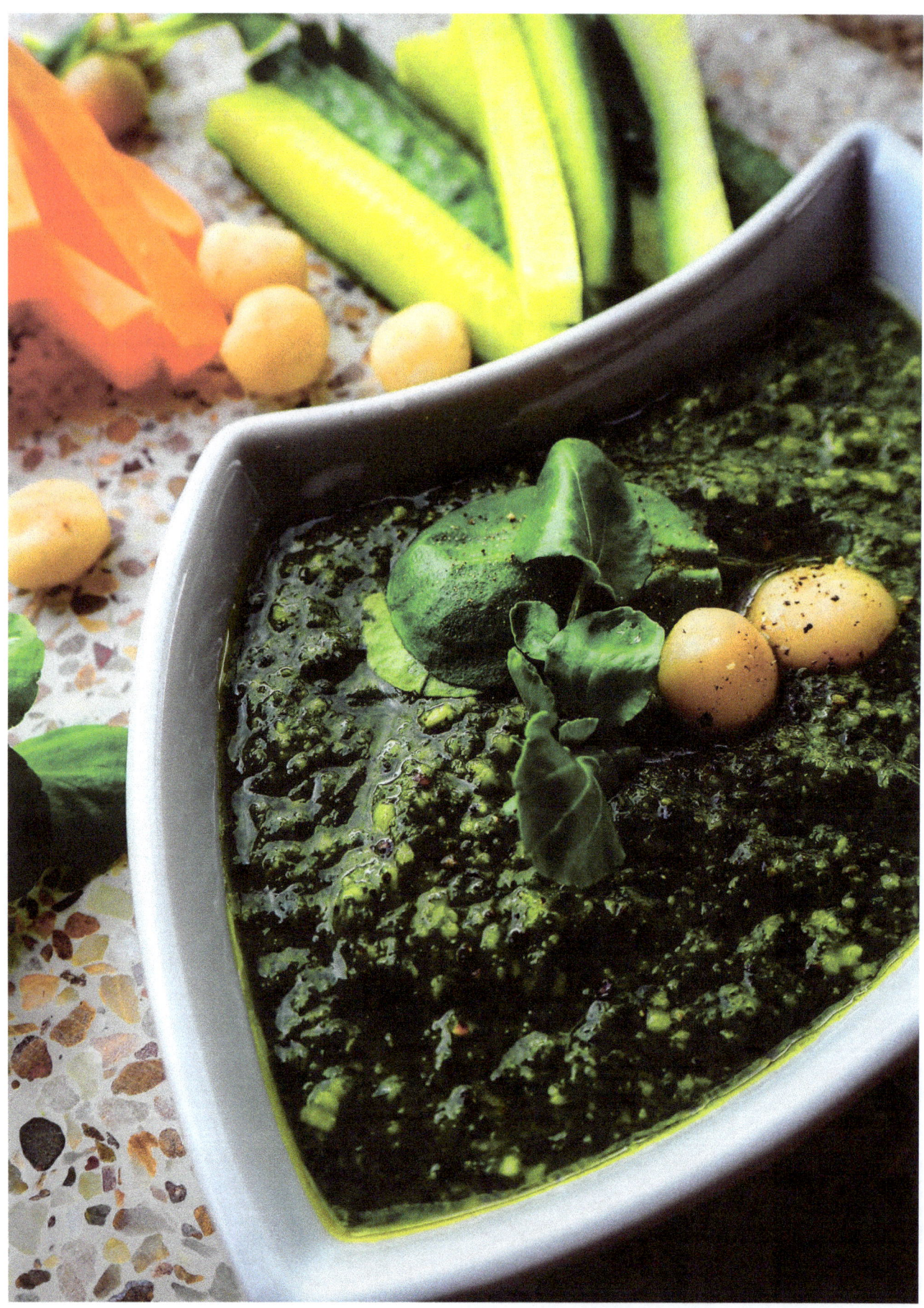

Herb Macadamia Pesto

Makes 2 average-sized jars

I love my pesto! Brimming with aromatic and gut-loving herbs, rich macadamias, and a kick from the lemon and garlic, you will want to have it in almost anything. It is such a flavourful and enriching condiment to have in sandwiches, on pizza, stirred through pasta, grilled fish, chicken and turkey dishes.

1-2 bunches flat-leaved parsley
1 bunch watercress, no stems (optional)
1-2 bunches basil leaves
1 bunch coriander leaves
A handful of mint (optional)
½ cup macadamia nuts
½ - ¾ teaspoon salt or more to taste
½ - 1 teaspoon pure maple syrup
1 ½ lemons, juiced
½ - 1 cup olive oil (add more if too dry)
2 tablespoon garlic-infused olive oil or to taste

Blitz all ingredients in a food processor until fairly smooth and the oil brings everything together in a thick paste.

Store in glass jars or freeze smaller portions in ziplock bags.

RECIPE NOTES

Pesto does require a lot of oil, so don't be afraid to give it some olive oil love.

Dad's Ginger Spring Onion Sauce

Makes 1 large jar or 2 medium-sized jars

Dad's ginger spring onion sauce is a harmonious accompaniment to roast chicken, barbecued pork ('char siew'), with rice or stir-fried noodles. The warming, peppery intensity of the ginger, together with the sweet and bitey flavour from the spring onions make this a match made in heaven.

500 g fresh ginger
2 spring onion sprigs (green part only)
½ cup olive oil
½ teaspoon salt

Wash the ginger and scrape the skin off with a small knife or teaspoon. Cut the ginger into small chunks and blend them in a food processor. Place the blended ginger into a heat-resistant bowl.

Wash and slice the green part of the spring onions into small pieces. Add them to the blended ginger.

In a small saucepan, heat up the olive oil for a few minutes (not at boiling point) and pour it into the blended ginger. Add salt to taste.

Store in a glass jar and consume within 1 week.

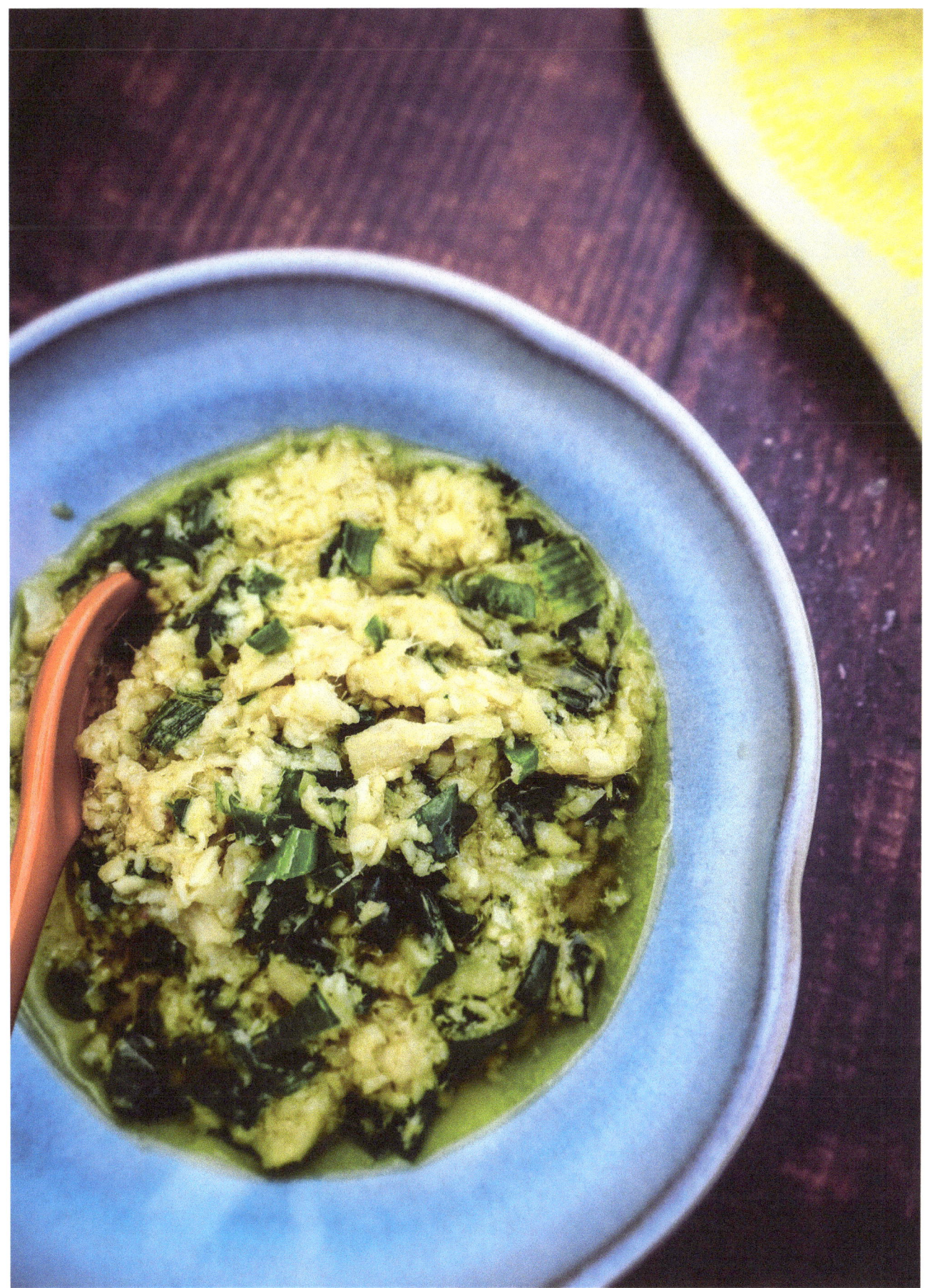

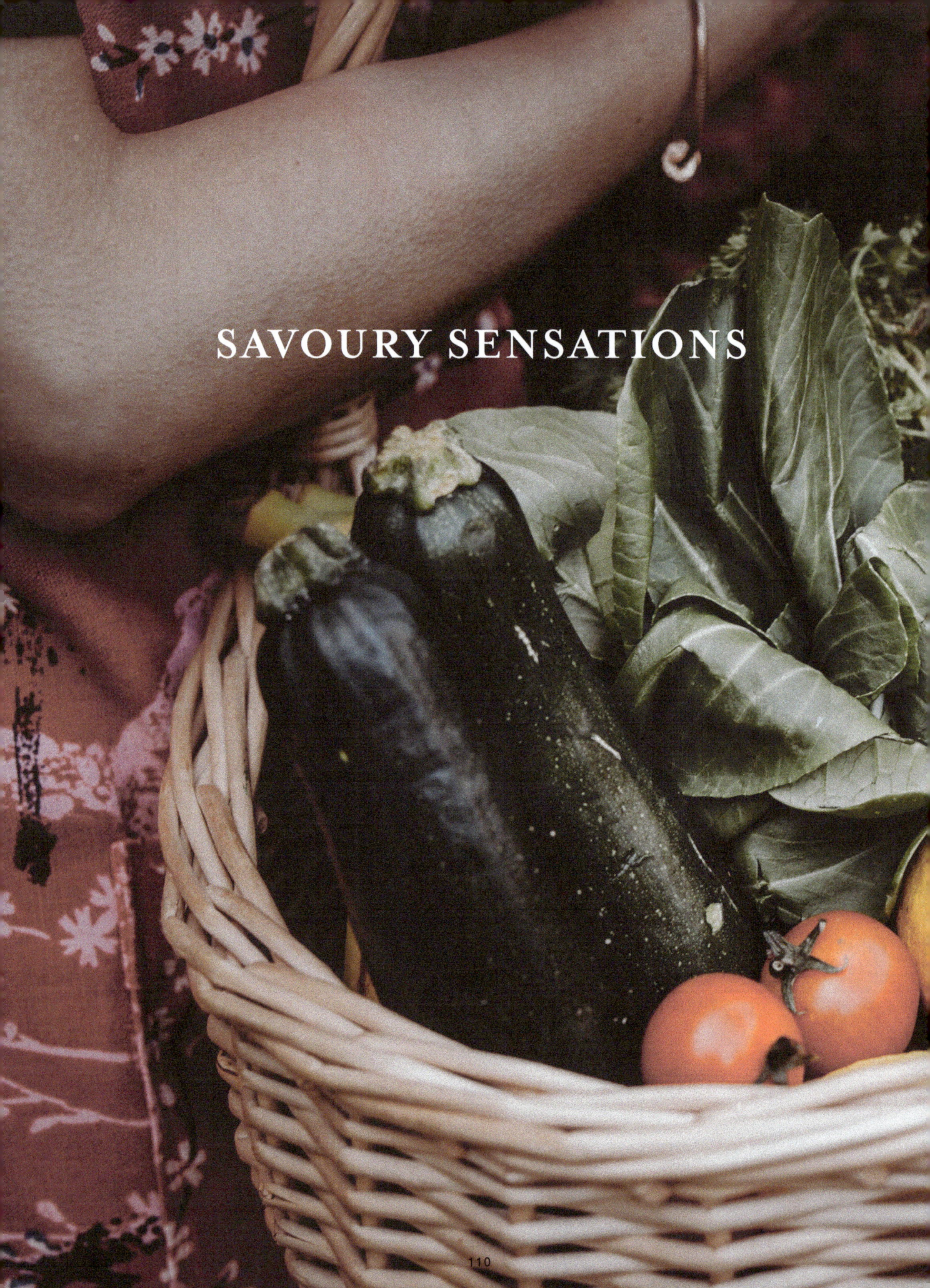

SAVOURY SENSATIONS

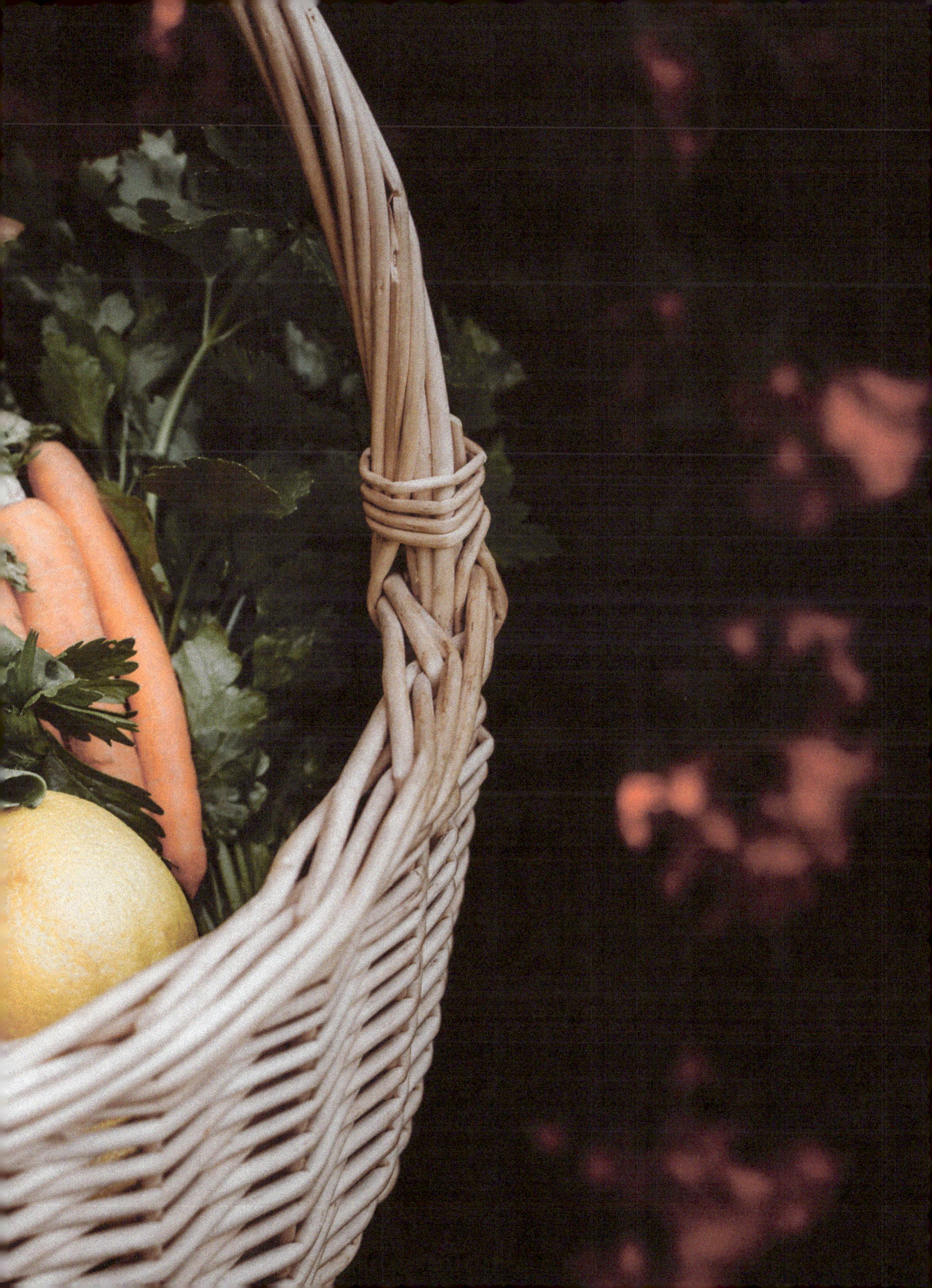

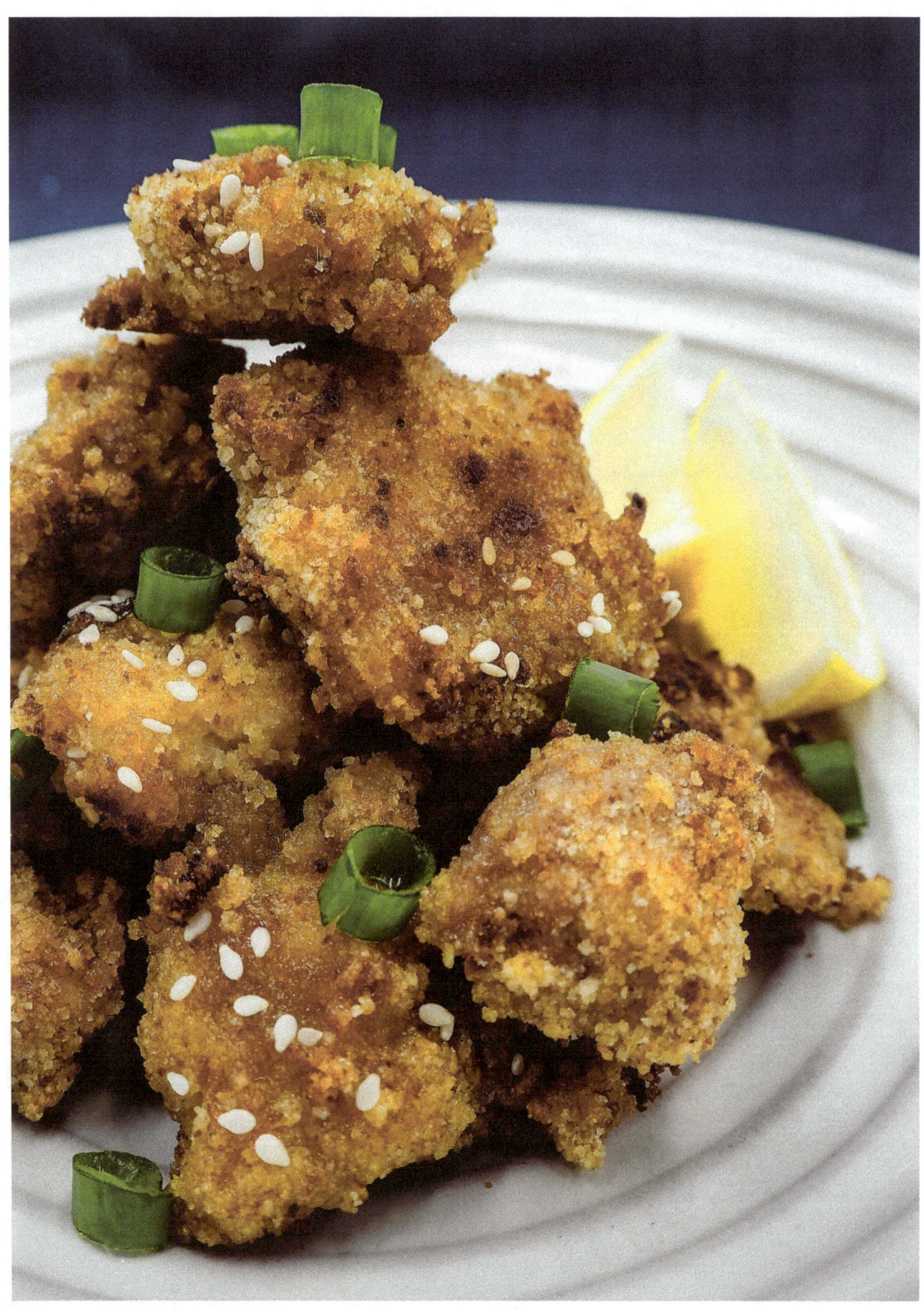

Baked Maple Lemon-Glazed Chicken

Serves 8-10 people

Your Friday night (or any weeknight) dinner is sorted with this twist to a honey lemon chicken; using maple syrup instead! Crispy baked chicken tossed in a sticky, sweet and sour maple lemon glaze, with notes of garlic and chives; this dish goes superbly well with rice and stir-fried vegetables.

1 kg skinless free-range chicken thigh fillets, cut into bite-sized pieces
1 ½ teaspoons salt or to taste
Pinch of cracked black pepper
3 large free-range eggs, beaten
2-3 cups gluten-free breadcrumbs or quinoa flakes

MAPLE LEMON GLAZE
⅓ cup pure maple syrup
1 tablespoon garlic-infused olive oil
1 tablespoon olive oil
Juice of ¾ - 1 lemon
½ teaspoon salt
1 tablespoon tapioca starch or arrowroot starch
½ cup water
2 spring onion sprigs (green part only) or 4 sprigs of chives
2 teaspoons sesame seeds

Preheat the oven to 200°c and line a baking tray. Season the chicken pieces with salt and pepper. Dip each piece of chicken into the beaten eggs and coat them with the breadcrumbs or quinoa flakes.

Spread the chicken pieces out on the baking tray and bake for 30 minutes, turning them over half way to ensure even browning and crispiness.

Just before the chicken comes out of the oven, combine all the ingredients for the glaze into a saucepan and heat on medium-high heat until simmering and thickened. Stir through the sesame seeds.

Once the chicken is ready, toss the chicken pieces (a few at a time), gently in the glaze and spread them out on the baking tray to prevent them from sticking to each other. Return the tray to the oven and bake for a further 5 minutes. Serve with rice and vegetables.

RECIPE NOTES

If you like, you can make additional glaze to pour over the chicken once served.

Salmon Sweet Potato Fritters

Makes 18 fritters

These fritters are satisfying and bursting with flavour. Packed with essential omega-3 and good oils from the salmon, plus loads of nutrients and fibre from the vegetables, these are great for a light lunch, served up with your favourite dairy-free aioli and a refreshing salad.

2 medium-sized sweet potatoes, steamed and mashed
370 g wild-caught salmon (2 medium-sized fillets)
1 large zucchini, shredded and juice squeezed
2 carrots, shredded
The rind of ½ lemon
2 tablespoons fresh parsley, chopped finely
Pinch of dried dill
2 teaspoons garlic-infused olive oil
½ teaspoon salt
1 free-range egg
¼ cup Gluten-Free Flour Blend — Option 1
¼ cup millet flour
Or
½ cup Gluten-Free Flour Blend — Option 2

Par-cook the salmon fillets by pan-frying or grilling them in some garlic-infused olive oil. Once cooked, remove the skin and flake the rest into pieces. In a mixing bowl, add all the ingredients together and mix thoroughly until a batter is formed.

Over medium heat, drizzle some olive oil in a frying pan and ladle about 4 tablespoons of batter each, frying 4 fritters at a time. Let them seal for about 2-3 minutes before flipping them over to seal the other side. Remove them from the pan once they are golden brown.

Serve immediately.

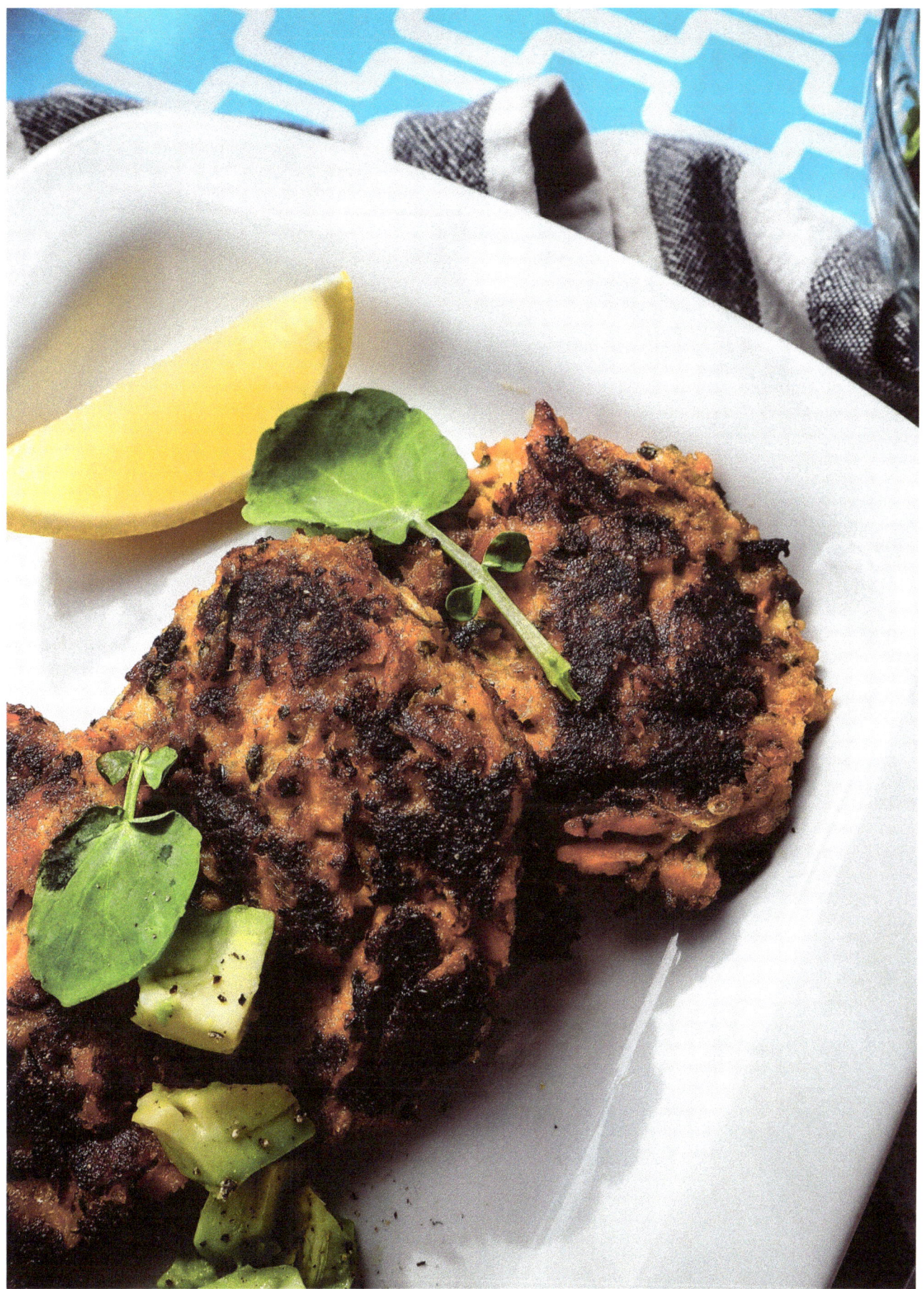

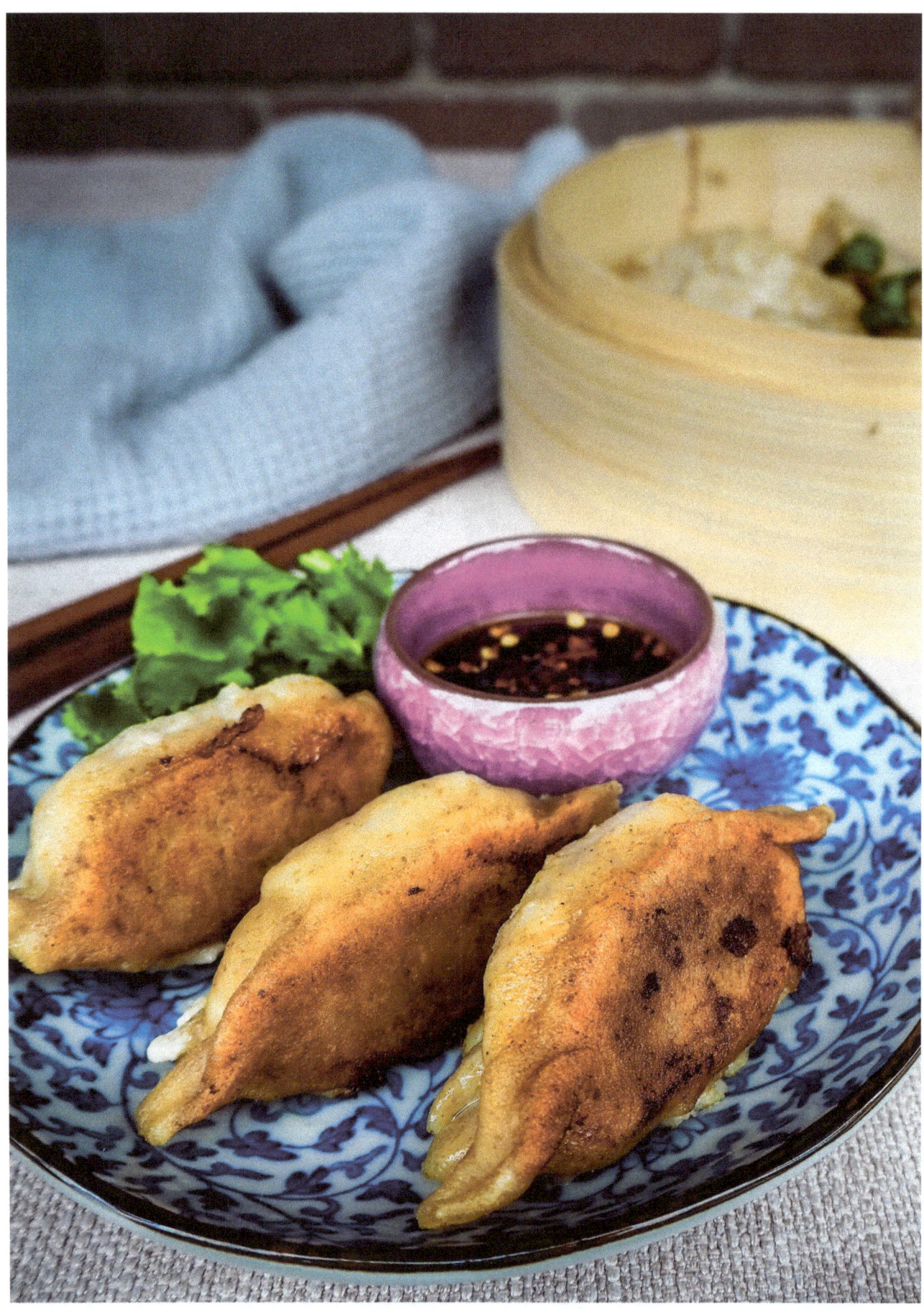

Pork & Chicken Pot Sticker Dumplings

Makes 42 dumplings

Time and time again, I would find myself standing outside my favourite dumpling restaurant, longing to devour a whole plate of dumplings once more. Crispy golden-brown skin, yet chewy without being gummy, encasing a juicy filling that oozes with flavour. I was determined to create this comforting classic — without the gluten! These dumplings are delightful and sure to impress your family and friends.

CHICKEN & PORK FILLING
500 g organic pork mince
500 g free-range chicken mince
2 carrots, shredded
6-7 chives or 3 spring onion sprigs (green part only), finely chopped
2 large handfuls coriander leaves
1 ¼ teaspoon salt or to taste
2 teaspoons pure maple syrup
2 tablespoons garlic-infused and ginger-infused olive oil*
1 tablespoon arrowroot starch
½ teaspoon lemon juice

DUMPLING DOUGH
1 ½ cups brown rice flour
½ cup millet flour
¾ cup tapioca starch
2 tablespoons golden flaxseed meal
½ cup glutinous rice flour
1 ⅓ cups & 4 tablespoons boiling water
4 teaspoons olive oil
Extra brown rice flour for dusting

FILLING & ASSEMBLING
Make the dumpling filling the day before by adding all ingredients together in a bowl. Mix well to combine. If you like, microwave a tablespoon's worth of filling to test if it is appropriately seasoned.

Across two lined trays, shape about 1 ½ tablespoons of filling into quenelles, leaving small gaps in between each ball. You should have 42 portions ready. The remainder of the mix can be used to make pork chicken balls or whatever you desire. Cling wrap the 2 trays, and place in the freezer overnight.

The following day, make the dough for the dumpling wrappers. Place all ingredients into a mixing bowl, add boiling water and mix until it comes together to form a dough.

Use your hands to knead the dough in the bowl until a smooth ball is formed. Place dough onto a dusted board and knead for a further 2 minutes.

Remove the two trays carrying the frozen filling portions from the freezer and set aside.

Divide the dough into approximately 42 pieces. The easiest way is to first divide the dough into half, roll one half into a long roll (about 2 cm in diameter), and roughly 40 cm long. Cut into 21 pieces, each about 3 cm long (it should look like pieces of gnocchi) and set aside on a plate. Cover them with a damp tea towel to prevent moisture loss. Repeat with the other half of the dough. You should end up with 42 pieces of the same size.

Pork & Chicken Pot Sticker Dumplings Continued —

*GARLIC & GINGER-INFUSED OLIVE OIL

Pan-fry a thumb-sized ginger piece and 2 cloves of garlic (both sliced thinly) in ¼ cup olive oil until both the ginger and garlic are slightly brown and fragrant. Let the oil cool down and store in a glass or ceramic container.

OR

Pan-fry a thumb-sized ginger piece (thinly sliced) in ¼ cup garlic-infused olive oil until the ginger pieces are slightly brown and fragrant. Let the oil cool down and pour in a glass or ceramic container.

Use 2 tablespoons of the infused-oil in the meat filling mixture.

To assemble, lightly dust a clean board with brown rice flour and begin to smooth out each piece with a rolling pin to form a disc shape, about 7 cm in diameter. Place rolled out dough onto your palm and put the frozen filling onto the centre. Dab some water around the rim of the dough wrapper. Join two opposite sides of the wrapper together and start to fold pleats along the wrapper, making sure it is sealed well and there are no holes or gaps in the wrapper.

Repeat the process for all dough wrappers. As you go, place finished dumplings under a damp tea towel across two trays to prevent them from drying out and cracking.

PAN-FRYING

Add 2-4 tablespoons of olive oil into a non-stick pan (one with a cover). Place dumplings flat side down and allow them to sear to a light golden brown.

Once they start to brown (about 6 minutes), add about ¼ cup of boiling water to the pan, avoiding pouring directly on the dumplings and close the lid. Cook on low to medium heat for 5 minutes.

Remove the lid and let the remaining water evaporate. Cook for a further 6 minutes to allow them to crispen and continue browning up on the bottom.

Dish out the dumplings onto a serving plate, with the golden brown flat side facing up.

RECIPE NOTES

You can freeze pre-cooked dumplings by wrapping the tray in cling wrap and placing in the freezer until wrappers are completely frozen. Remove and place in ziplock bags or in airtight containers. If cooking frozen dumplings, it takes approximately 8 minutes to brown before adding boiling water. Once water is added, the rest of the cooking process will take about 10-15 minutes.

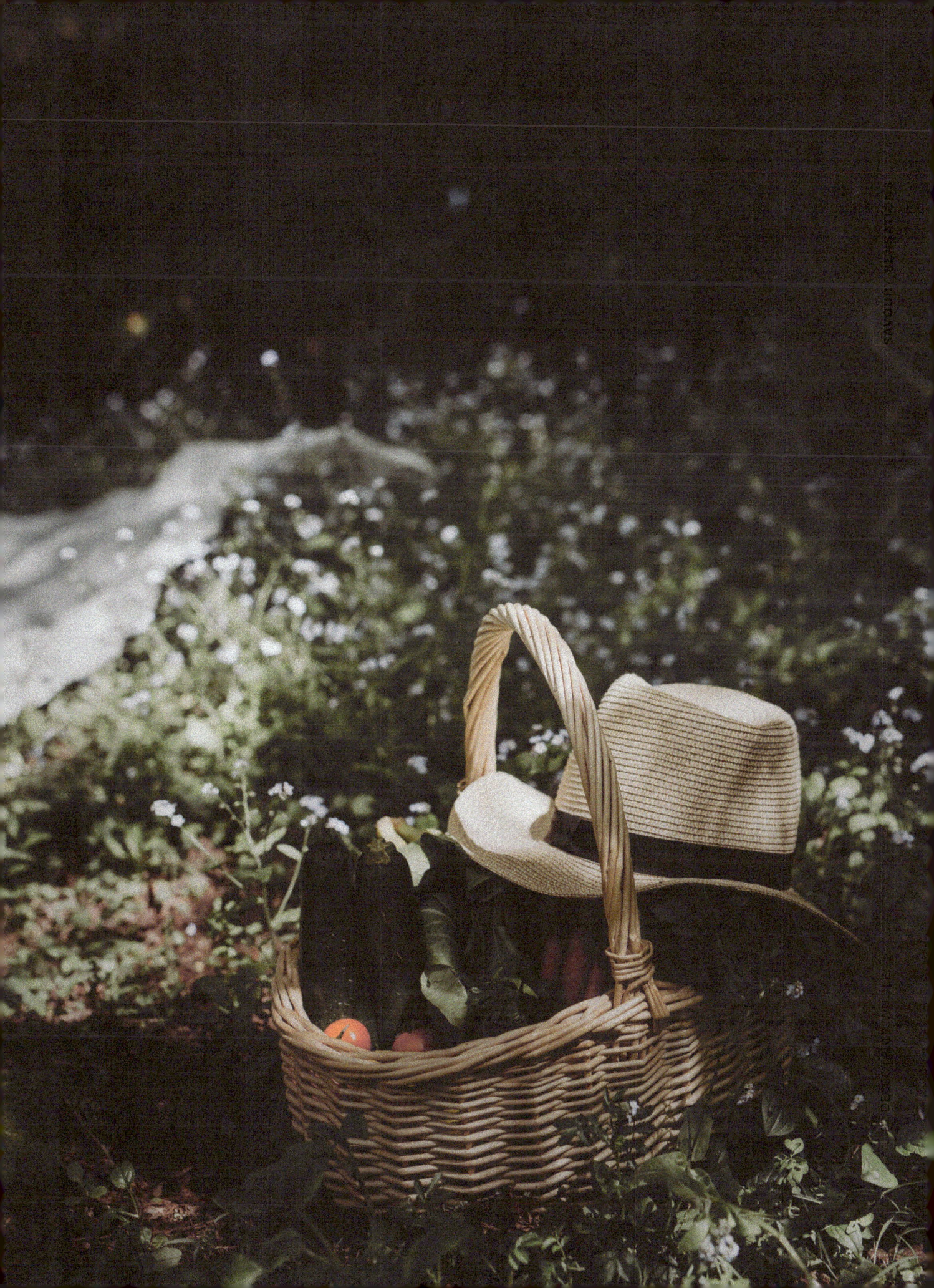

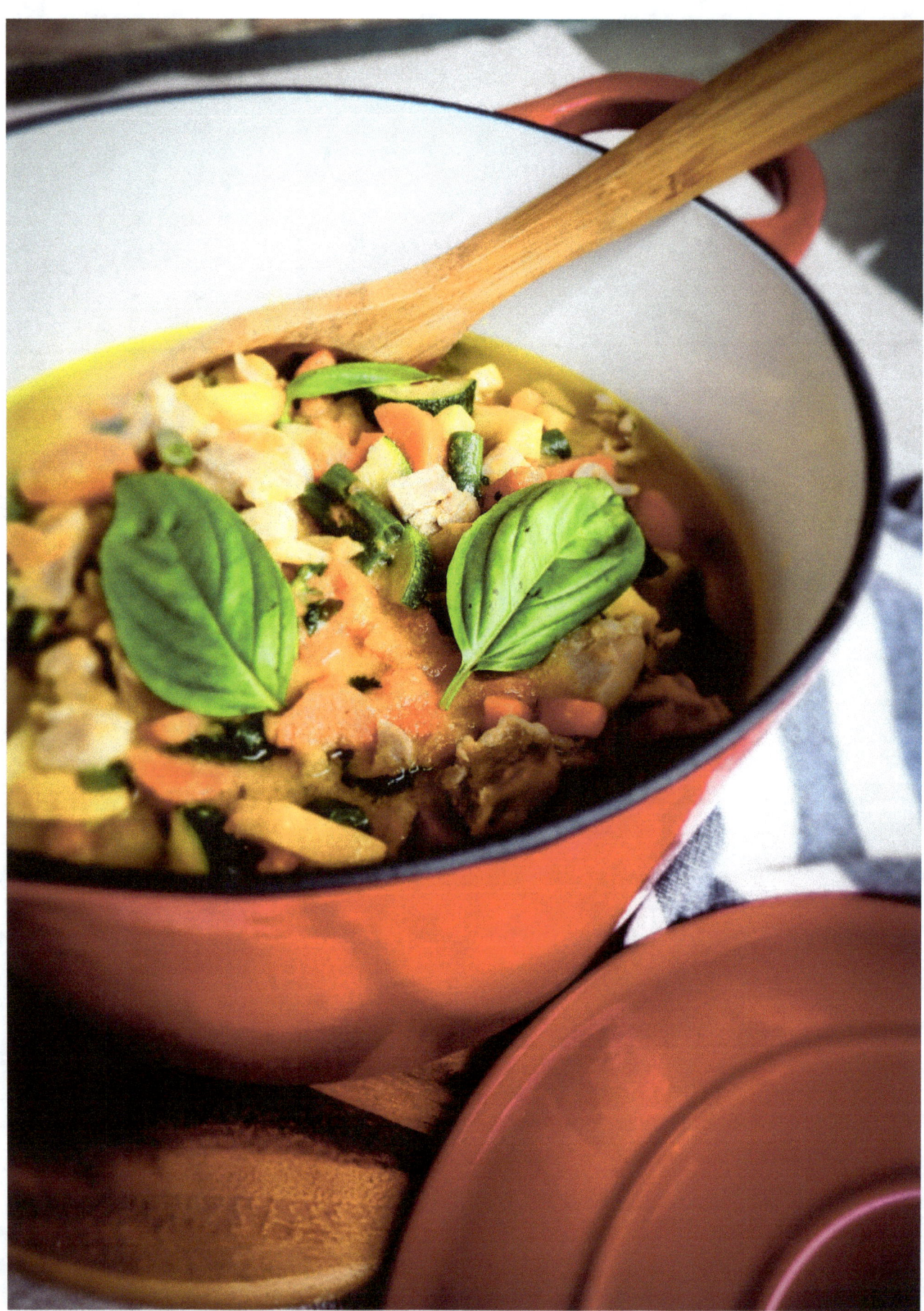

Creamy Thai Chicken Curry

Makes 6-8 serves

This flavoursome and comforting chicken curry, infused with Thai flavours, takes me back to dining at a Thai restaurant. The distinctive aroma and taste of the kaffir lime leaves sing out when they are teamed up with fresh basil and coriander. Together, the coconut cream and sweet potato provide an irresistible creaminess to this dish, which pairs perfectly with freshly steamed basmati rice and a side of green vegetables.

4 kaffir lime leaves
3 spring onion sprigs (green part only) or chives, sliced finely
Handful of basil leaves
Handful of coriander leaves
1 tablespoon julienne ginger
1-2 tablespoons olive oil
1 tablespoon garlic-infused olive oil
3 medium-sized carrots, sliced
2 medium-sized zucchinis, sliced
A handful of green beans, chopped
½ medium-sized sweet potato, cubed
6 free-range boneless chicken thigh fillets, cut into bite-size pieces
½ cup coconut milk or cream
1 cup water
1 ½ teaspoons salt, or to taste
2 tablespoons pure maple syrup
Pinch of cracked pepper
A squeeze of lemon juice
1 ½ tablespoons arrowroot starch

Prepare all your ingredients before you begin the cooking process.

On medium heat, drizzle olive oil and garlic-infused olive oil in a deep frying pan. Add in the ginger and fry until golden and fragrant. Add in the kaffir lime leaves, sliced carrots and sweet potato and stir fry for 2 minutes. Add in a dash of water, cover and let simmer for about 8 minutes or until the vegetables begin to soften.

Add in chicken pieces and spring onion and stir through. Add salt, maple syrup, cracked pepper, coconut milk and water and continue stirring. Cover and let it simmer for around 5 minutes until the chicken is half cooked.

Add in the zucchini and beans and stir to combine. Cover and let it simmer for another 5 minutes until the chicken is cooked all the way through and the zucchini and beans are just cooked. All the natural juices from the chicken and vegetables have now created a beautiful creamy curry, together with the coconut milk.

Add in the coriander, basil leaves, a squeeze of lemon juice and arrowroot starch. Stir to combine and taste, adding more salt if needed.

The curry should be bubbling away at a steady pace. Turn the fire off and serve.

RECIPE NOTES

This curry is best served with steamed rice and green leafy vegetables. If you can handle more spice, add some chilli or more pepper to the mix.

Frittata

Serves 8 people

This vibrant eggy sensation is a nutritious, protein-packed option for lunch or dinner. Loaded with vegetable goodness, eggs, and little accents of naturally wood-smoked bacon, it is a light and deliciously satisfying one-pot meal you will want to have as a staple in your home.

2 large or 3 small carrots, grated
1 medium-sized sweet potato (approximate 1 cup), grated
1 large or 2 small zucchinis, grated
3 strips nitrate-free, naturally wood-smoked shortcut bacon (rind removed), diced
6-7 free-range eggs
⅓ cup unsweetened almond milk
Handful of freshly chopped parsley and basil
Fresh or dried rosemary, thyme and oregano or whatever herbs you prefer
3 spring onion sprigs or chives
½ teaspoon salt
Pinch of cracked pepper
1 cup Gluten-Free Flour Blend — Option 1
2 teaspoons baking powder
½ cup olive oil
1 tablespoon garlic-infused olive oil for frying bacon pieces

TOPPING
½ cup grated cheese (dairy-free, low-lactose or lactose-free)
5 cherry tomatoes, sliced into quarters

Grate all vegetables. In a separate bowl, whisk eggs together with chopped fresh or dried herbs. Add salt, pepper, ½ cup olive oil, milk, and whisk to mix.

Pan fry bacon pieces in some garlic-infused olive oil and a little olive oil. Fry till bacon pieces are golden brown. Add grated vegetables and bacon pieces plus the residual oil from the pan into the egg mixture.

Add in the flour and mix well until a thick batter forms. Pour the batter into a 20-30 cm lined skillet (double line the skillet with baking paper to prevent the bottom from burning).

Place chopped cherry tomatoes on the top, followed by the grated cheese. Cover the skillet and let it cook on the stove on a low heat for 30-45 minutes. At the halfway mark, remove the lid to let the steam out so it doesn't overheat and cause the eggs to expand too quickly, as this will result in an uneven surface. Repeat this at the 30-minute mark. Place the lid back on to finish the cooking process.

Once an inserted fork comes out clean from the middle, turn the heat off. Let it cool for a bit before slicing. Serve with a side salad.

RECIPE NOTES

If you have a gas stovetop, ensure that your pan is placed on a smaller-sized burner as this will allow the frittata to cook more consistently and evenly, without burning the bottom crust.

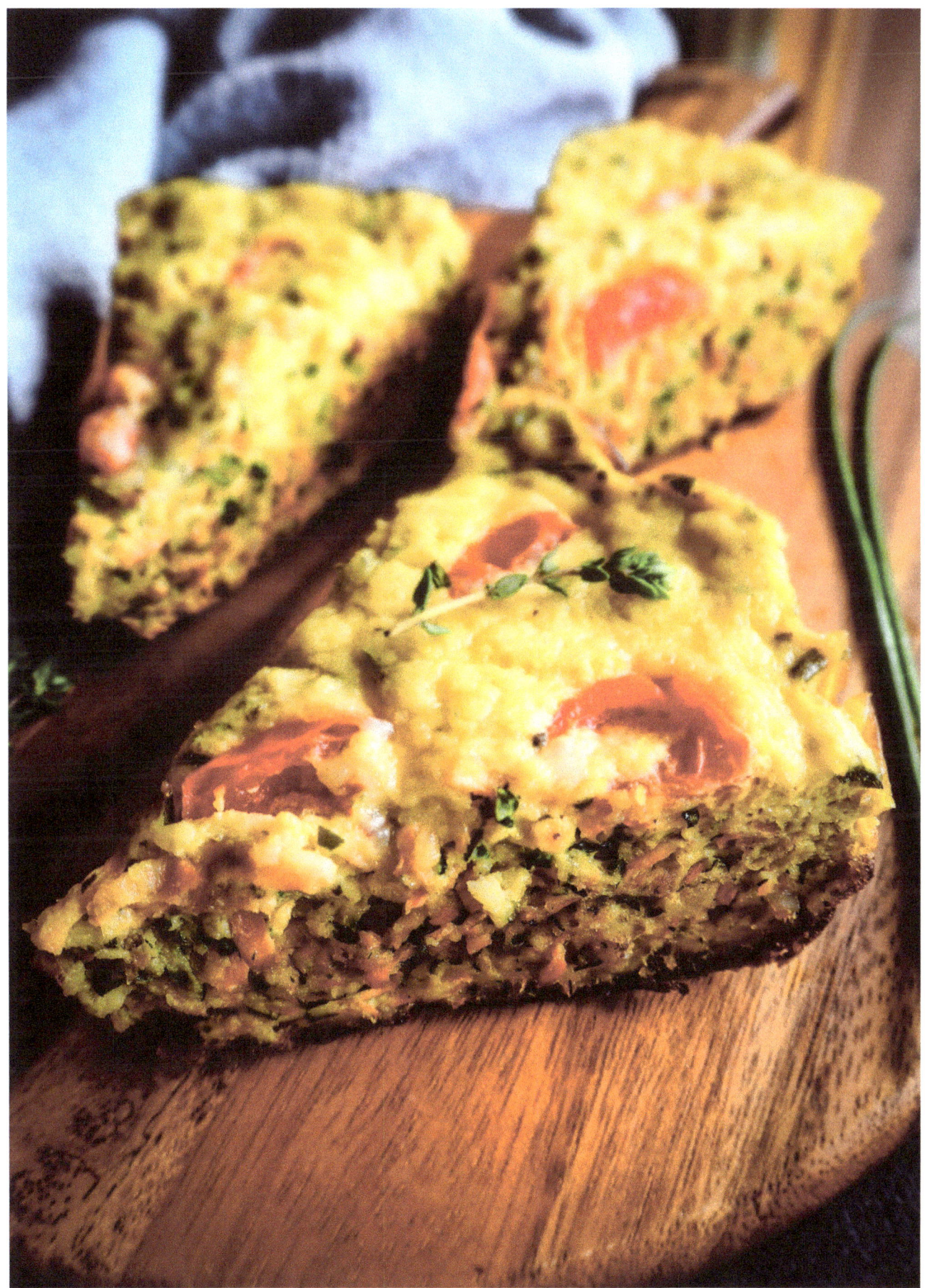

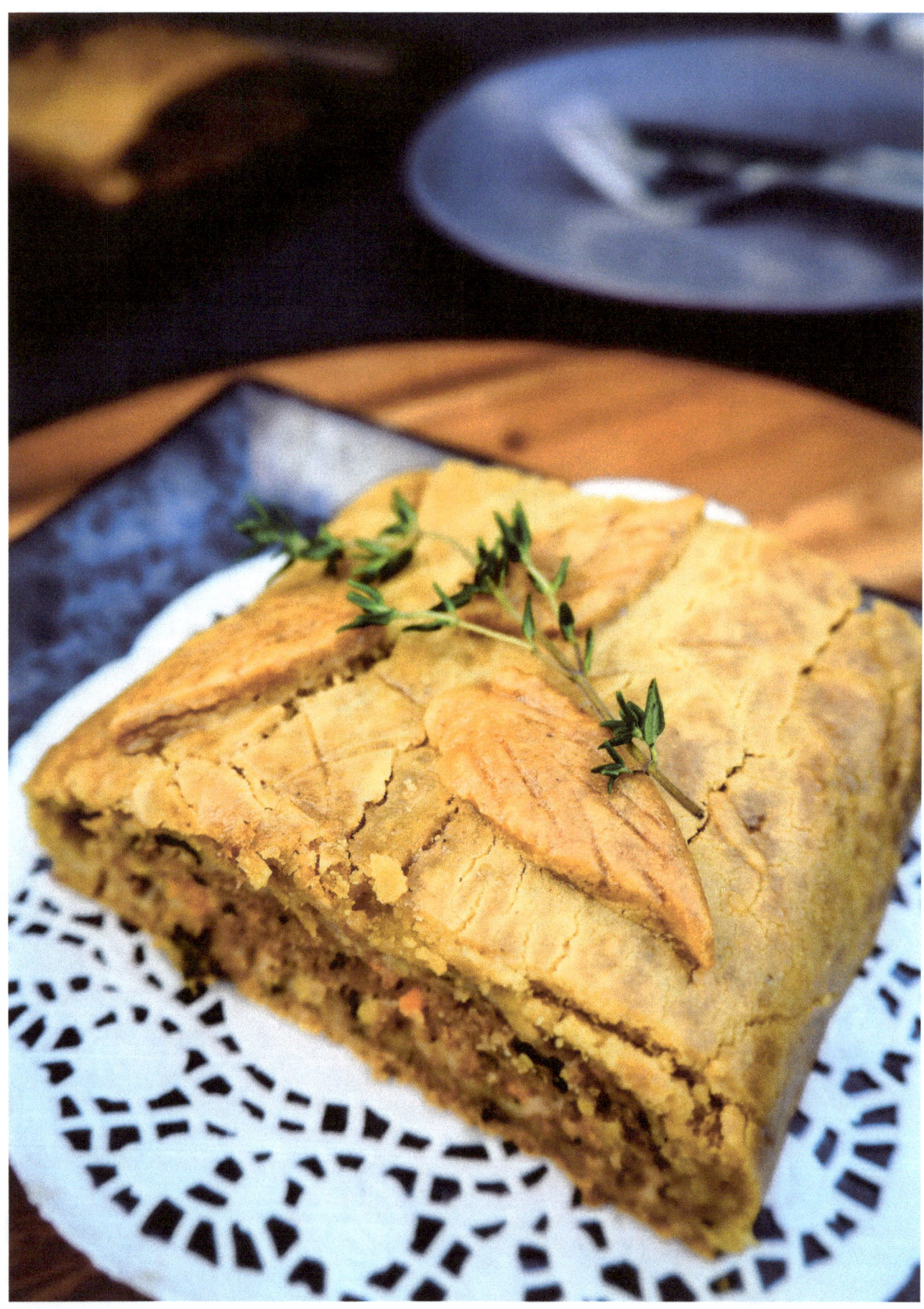

Pork & Turkey Sausage Rolls

Makes 3 large rolls or 12 small rolls

These mouth-watering and flavourful sausage rolls make for an exciting picnic lunch treat. Succulent meat enveloped by flaky shortcrust pastry, accompanied by a fresh salad — this will become a well-loved family recipe for years to come.

SHORTCRUST PASTRY
¼ cup cassava flour
¼ cup sorghum flour
½ cup tapioca starch
½ cup millet flour
½ cup glutinous rice flour
½ cup quinoa flour
1 teaspoon golden flaxseed meal
2 teaspoons hot water
½ teaspoon salt
1 teaspoon baking soda
1 teaspoon coconut sugar
1 teaspoon apple cider vinegar
125 g cold vegan butter, chopped
7 tablespoons iced-cold water

To make the shortcrust pastry, mix a teaspoon of the flaxseed meal with 2 teaspoons of hot water in a small bowl. Let it sit for 5 minutes and set aside.

In a food processor, blitz together the flours, salt, baking soda, coconut sugar, apple cider vinegar and vegan butter cubes until a fine crumb is achieved.

Transfer the mixture to a mixing bowl, and add the flaxseed meal gel and iced water, a tablespoon at a time until it forms a dough. It should be similar to playdough consistency. Knead until smooth. Cling wrap the dough and rest in the fridge for 30-40 minutes.

While the dough is resting in the fridge, make the filling. Combine all of the ingredients together and mix thoroughly. Place back in the fridge to keep cool until the dough is ready to be rolled out.

ASSEMBLY
Preheat the oven to 175°c and line two baking trays. Divide the dough into half. Cover the other half to avoid it drying out and set aside. Place the first half of the dough in the middle of a silicone mat and then put a piece of baking paper on top of the dough. Using a rolling pin, roll out the dough until it is 3 mm thick, 29 cm long and 24 cm wide.

Upon removing the baking paper, spoon the cold meat filling onto the rolled out dough and flatten slightly, about 8 cm wide and 20 cm long so that the filling nearly meets the edges of the dough. Carefully use the silicone mat to bend and guide the dough to roll over the filling until it meets the other side of the dough.

Pork & Turkey Sausage Rolls Continued —

MEAT FILLING
500 g organic pork mince
500 g turkey mince
2 sage leaves
3 fresh thyme sprigs or ¼ teaspoon dried thyme
4 spring onion sprigs (green part only) or chives, chopped finely
Handful of fresh parsley, chopped or ¼ teaspoon dried parsley
1 free-range egg
2 tablespoons garlic-infused olive oil and olive oil
½ sweet potato, peeled and diced (optional)
1 zucchini, grated and squeezed (optional)
1 carrot, grated (optional)
¼ cup gluten-free breadcrumbs
1 ½ teaspoons salt
Pinch of cracked pepper
2 teaspoons pure maple syrup
1 teaspoon apple cider vinegar
2 tablespoons arrowroot starch

1 egg, beaten for the egg wash

Cut off any excess dough. Keeping the edges unsealed, place the sausage roll on the lined baking tray. Repeat this process until the rest of the dough is finished. You will have some filling leftover, which would be perfect for meatballs.

Once all of the sausage rolls are on the baking trays, brush the tops of the sausage rolls with the egg wash. Using a fork, make small holes on the top of the pastry, so the steam can escape during baking.

Place in the oven and bake at 175°c for 20-30 minutes until the pastry is golden brown and cooked through. Let them cool on the baking trays for about 10 minutes before cutting and serving.

RECIPE NOTES

This recipe uses pork and turkey as the meats of choice. However, feel free to substitute with other meats such as lamb or beef, if preferred. The vegetables are an optional addition, but I find that they add great flavour and make these sausage rolls more nutritious. The method outlines making 3 large sausage rolls. However, if you are making 12 small rolls, the volume per roll would be different.

It is important to ensure that there are no cracks in the pastry when you roll it out, as the gaps will expand during cooking. These are freezer-friendly, too.

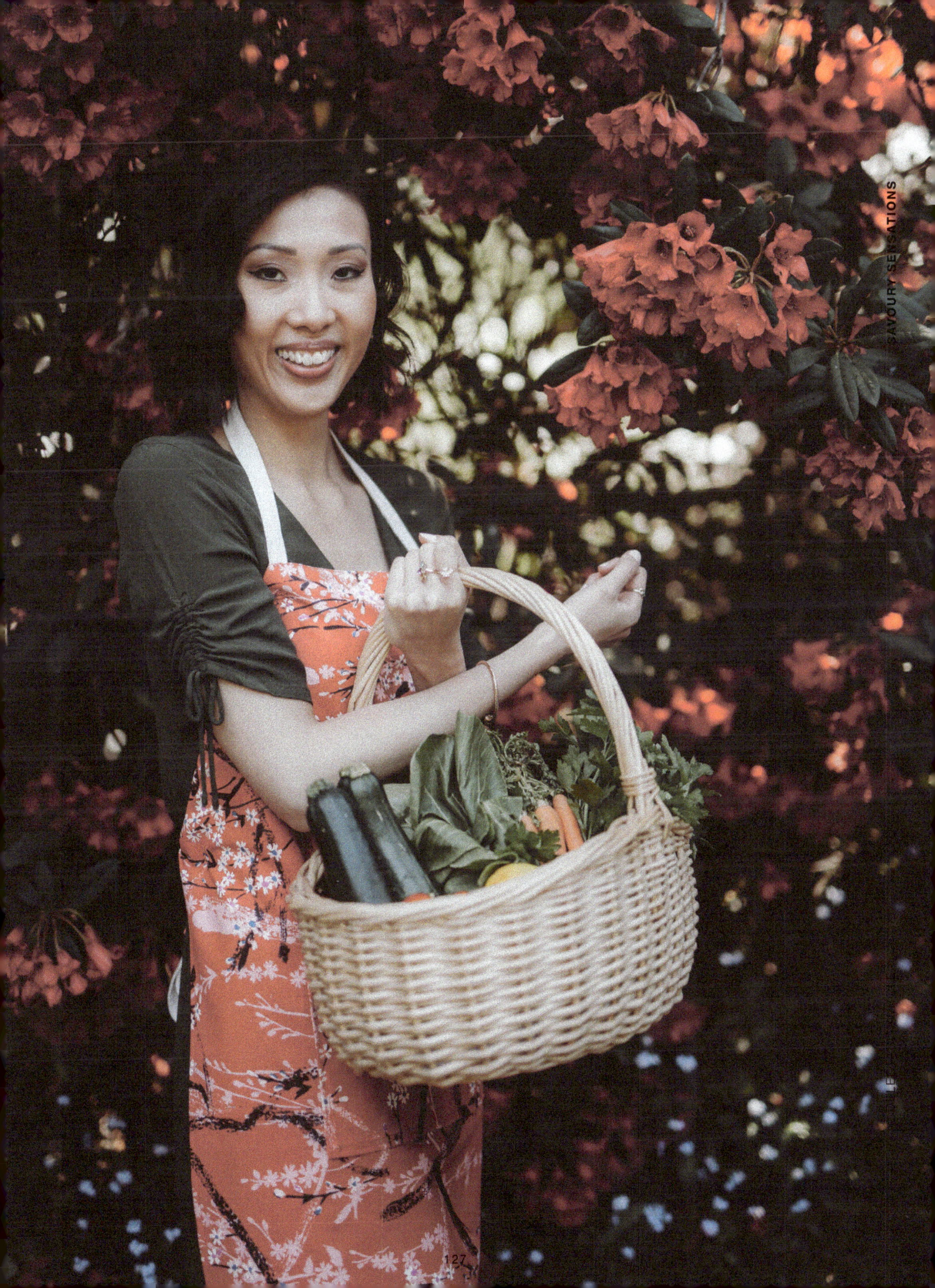

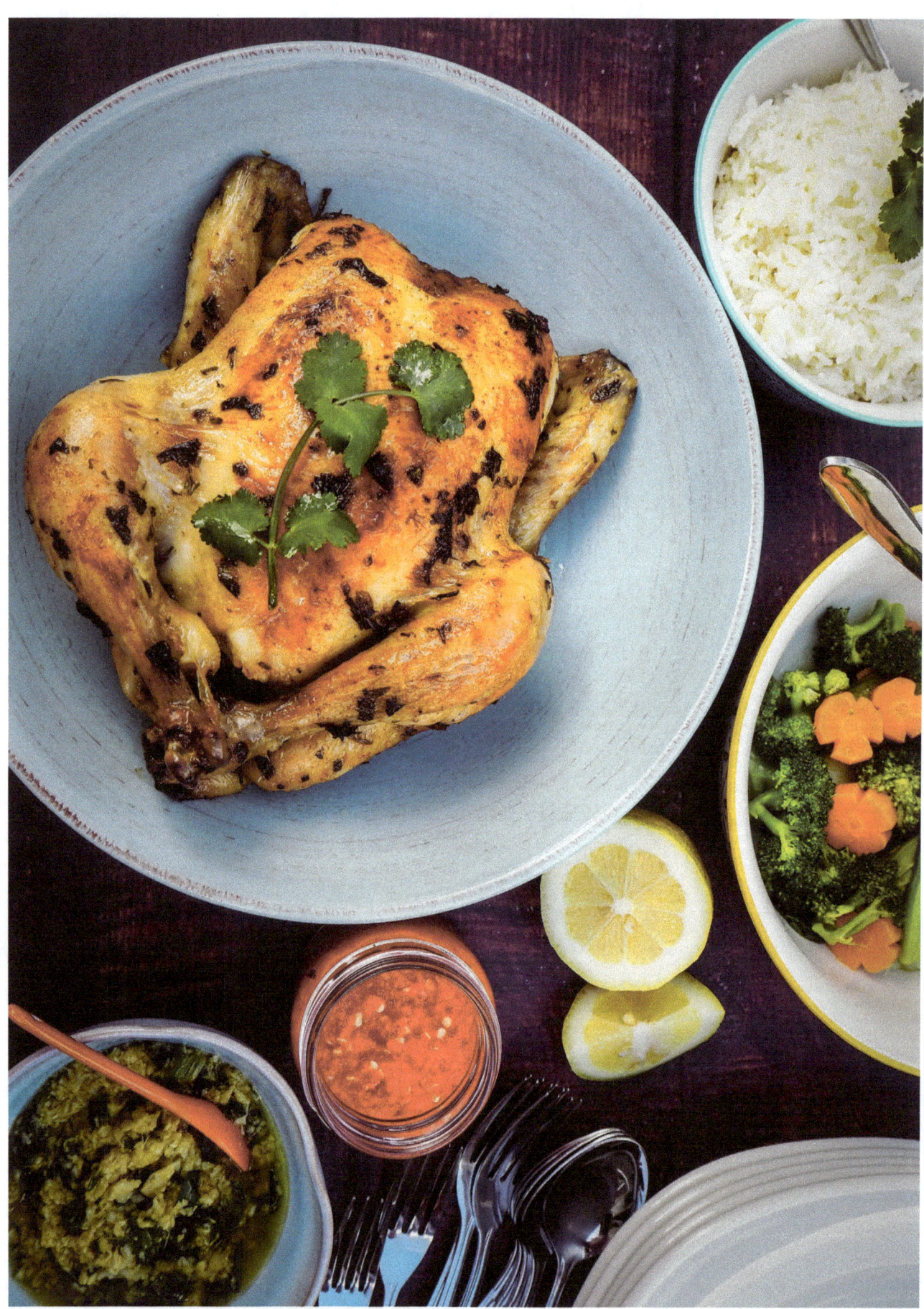

Roast Chicken Rice Feast

Serves 6 people

This would have to be one of my all-time favourite home-cooked meals, with a simple twist on the Hainanese-style chicken. It consists of my mum's succulent roast chicken, served with homemade chicken stock-infused rice, mixed vegetables and a side of my dad's ginger spring onion sauce. In my family, this is a traditional Chinese New Year family reunion meal and is usually made for birthdays or for just about any family gathering treat. This roast chicken rice feast will surely tantalise your tastebuds, with everyone wanting seconds!

MUM'S ROAST CHICKEN WITH CORIANDER
1 whole medium free-range organic chicken or 3-4 pieces of chicken Maryland, skin on
4 tablespoons garlic-infused olive oil
3 tablespoons pure maple syrup
2 teaspoons fresh grated ginger
Handful of coriander, chopped finely
1 tablespoon salt, or to taste

CHICKEN STOCK
8 free-range chicken drumsticks with skin on
2 medium carrots
3 slices of ginger
1 ½ teaspoon salt
2 litres filtered water

CHICKEN RICE
3 cups of chicken stock
Salt to taste
1 tablespoon garlic-infused olive oil
2 cups basmati rice (rinsed)

Clean the chicken and cut away unwanted fats. Dab the chicken dry with kitchen paper towels (including the inside of the bird).

Mix all ingredients in a bowl, and rub the seasoning all over the chicken including the inside. Place the chicken into a deeper baking tray, and tie both drumsticks together with cooking string. Let the chicken rest for an hour, covered in the fridge.

Preheat the oven to 210°c and roast the chicken for 1 hour 50 minutes, basting it with its own juices at the 1-hour mark and turning the tray around for even roasting.

Once an inserted skewer into the thigh area produces clear juice, remove the chicken from the oven, cover loosely with foil and let it rest for 30 minutes before serving.

Serve the roast chicken with the gravy juice from the roast pan.

CHICKEN STOCK
Boil the chicken stock for 1 hour until all the flavours have infused together. Using this stock, make the chicken rice.

CHICKEN RICE
In a large saucepan, rinse 2 cups of basmati rice and add 3 cups of the chicken stock to it. Add 2 teaspoons of garlic-infused olive oil for added flavour.

On medium to high heat and with the lid on, bring the rice to a boil. At boiling point, leave the lid ajar to prevent the rice from boiling over. Reduce to low heat, letting the rice simmer for about 15-20 minutes until fluffy and cooked.

Serve with ginger sauce (see Dad's Ginger Spring Onion Sauce recipe on page 108) and stir-fry mixed vegetables.

Crackling Roast Pork Belly

Serves 4 people

The satisfying crunch of crispy, crackling skin on a juicy, tender pork belly is an absolute crowd-pleaser and will have them wanting more! This may look overwhelming, but trust me, it is super easy and well worth the effort.

- 1 kg pork belly (free-range or organic is best)
- 2 tablespoons pink Himalayan fine salt (for seasoning the meat)
- 1 teaspoon five-spice powder (optional - considered high-histamine)
- 2 rice bowls regular table salt (for covering the pork skin)

Preheat the oven to 180°C. Turn the pork belly with skin side down. Slit the meat lengthwise without cutting all the way through. Make two slits if the piece of meat is wider. This will determine where you will cut the meat after it is cooked.

Mix the dry ingredients in a small bowl and marinate the meat, including the inside of the slitted part of the meat.

Turn the pork belly, skin side up. Wipe away any seasoning or moisture on the pork skin with a paper towel. Ensure that the pork skin is very dry.

Place the pork belly on a wire rack that fits inside a deep baking tray, lined with foil. Spread a generous layer of table salt (about ½ to 1 ½ cm thick), covering the entire surface of the skin (don't worry, this won't make the meat too salty - it is expected that some of the salt will fall into the tray).

Pour about 1 litre of hot boiling water into the baking tray (about 1 ½ cm deep), taking extra care not to wet the pork. Gently place the baking tray into the oven (middle rack) and roast at 180°C for 45 minutes.

The steam from the water will cause the salt to draw moisture from the skin, while the meat slowly roasts. The salt will become a stiff layer which can be removed easily with a pair of tongs after 45 minutes.

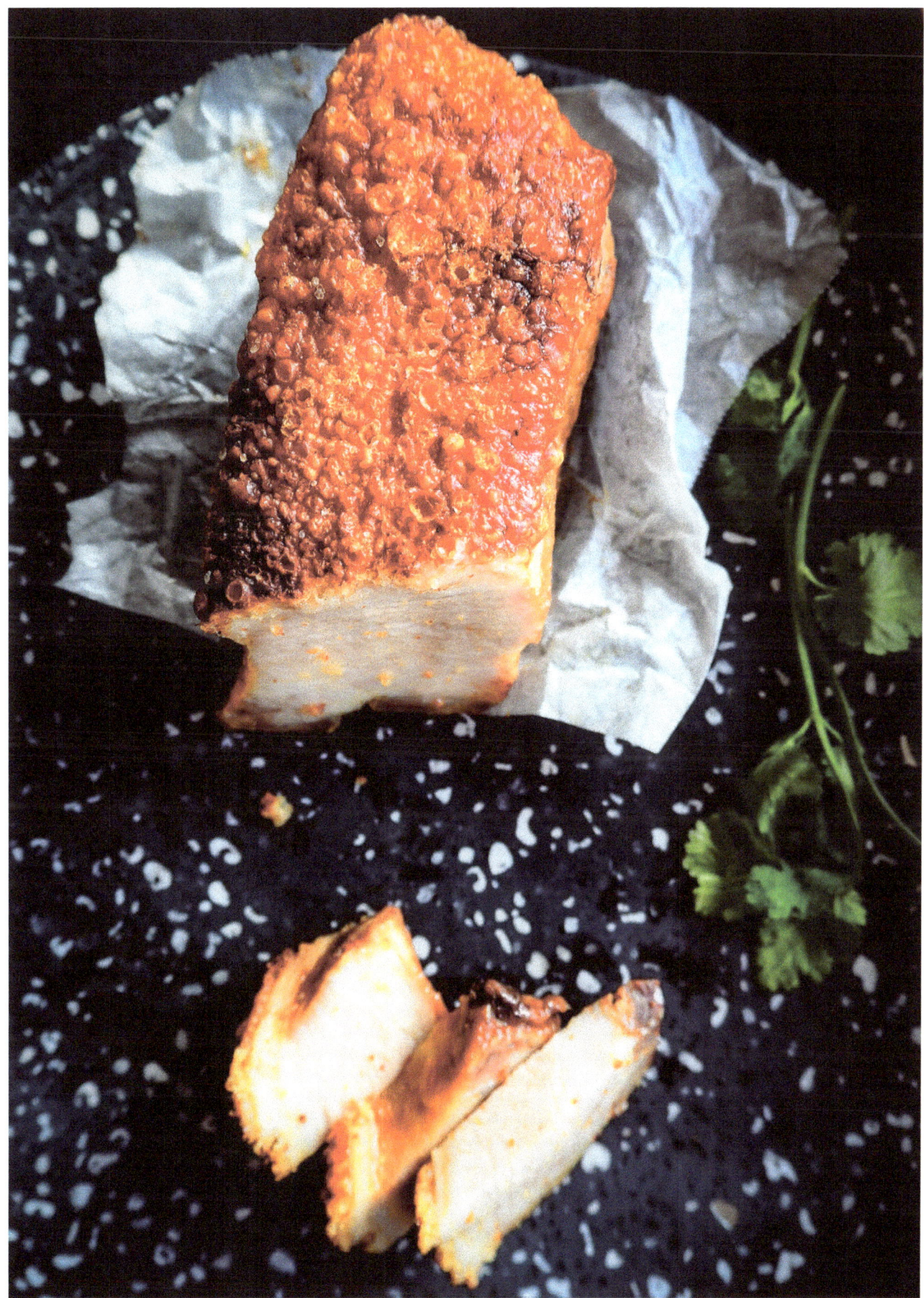

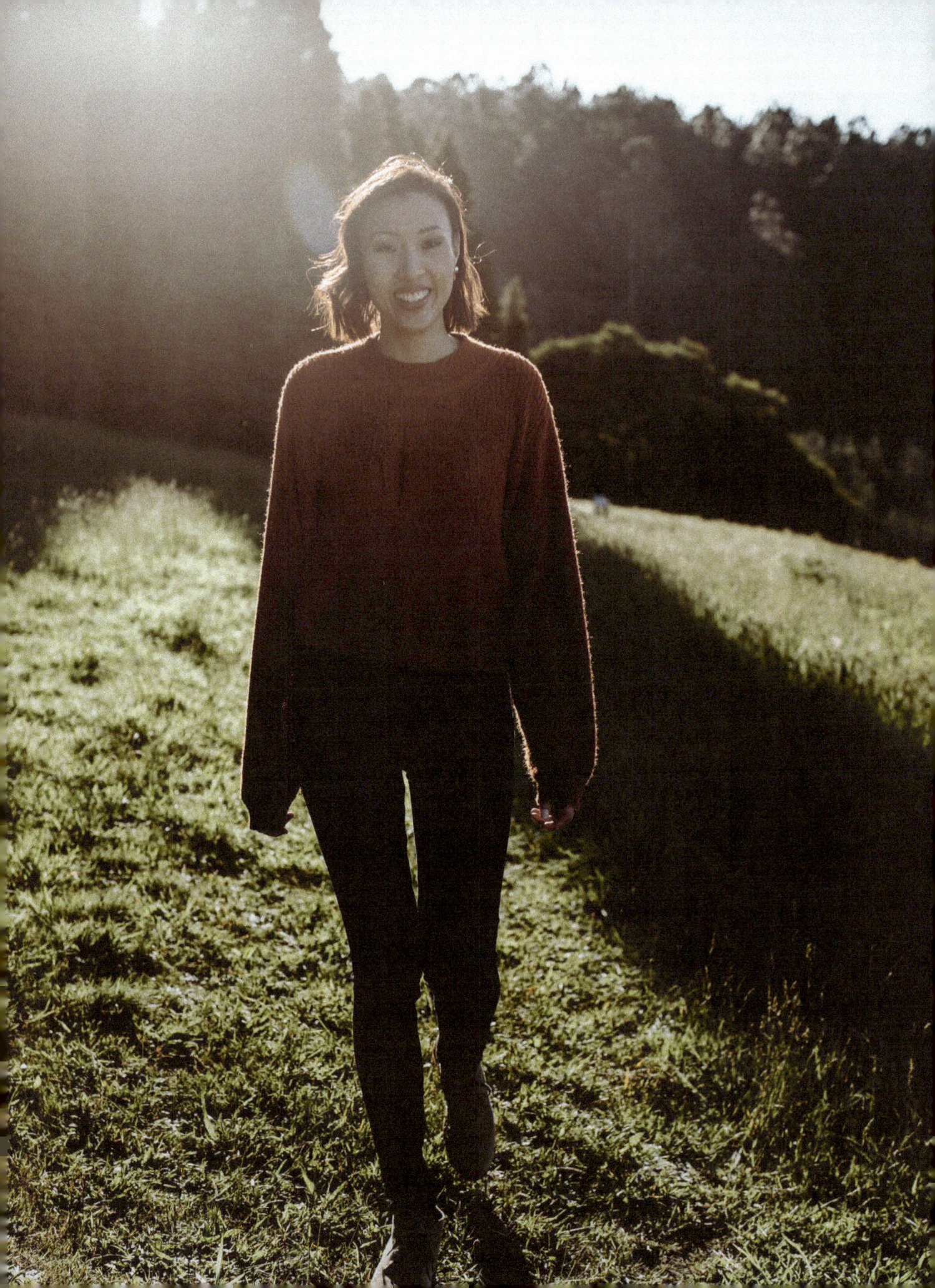

Crackling Roast Pork Belly Continued —

After the layer of salt is removed, increase the oven temperature to 240°c and return the pork into the oven to continue roasting for 20-30 minutes. Once cooked, allow the pork to sit for 15 minutes to rest.

To cut the crackling pork belly, turn the meat over with the skin side down. Find the slit made earlier, and push the knife down firmly, cutting all the way through. You should hear the crackling of the skin. Continue to slice the pork into smaller pieces by placing the strip of pork on its side and slide the knife firmly through the skin and meat.

RECIPE NOTES

It is best to get a good quality piece of pork belly from your local butcher. Ask for a piece that weighs around 1 kg and has a relatively even distribution of fat to meat ratio.

Crackling roast pork can be served with a variety of dishes: plain steamed rice and vegetables, green salad, dry or soupy noodles, or with chicken rice (see Roast Chicken Rice Feast recipe on page 129).

Vegetable Soup

Makes 8-10 serves

A well-rounded and wholesome meal, this warming soup is filled with immune-boosting vegetables, brimming with flavour and freshness. The coconut milk and ginger add a layer of depth and richness to the soup. Slow down and curl up with a bowl of this nutritious goodness, guaranteed to satisfy on cold days.

4 large carrots, sliced into medium-sized cubes
1 large orange sweet potato, sliced into medium-sized cubes
1 ½ cups sliced butternut pumpkin (equivalent to ¼ of an average-sized pumpkin)
1 medium-sized zucchini, diced into medium-sized cubes
1 teaspoon-sized knob of ginger, sliced
1 ½ teaspoons salt, or to taste
1 teaspoon garlic-infused olive oil
¼ cup pure organic coconut cream or milk
12 cups filtered water

Add all ingredients into an 8-litre stainless steel stockpot. Cover with the lid and heat on high until the soup begins to boil.

Turn it down to low-medium heat and simmer for about 1 ½ hours, checking occasionally to see if the vegetables have softened. Once the vegetables are all soft, turn the fire off and blitz the soup mixture with a stick mixer until the soup has reached a smooth consistency. Add more water depending on preferred thickness and adjust seasoning according to preference.

Garnish with fresh chopped parsley and a dash of cracked pepper.

RECIPE NOTES

To freeze portions, spoon soup into glass containers and freeze. Reheat over the stove or in a microwave.

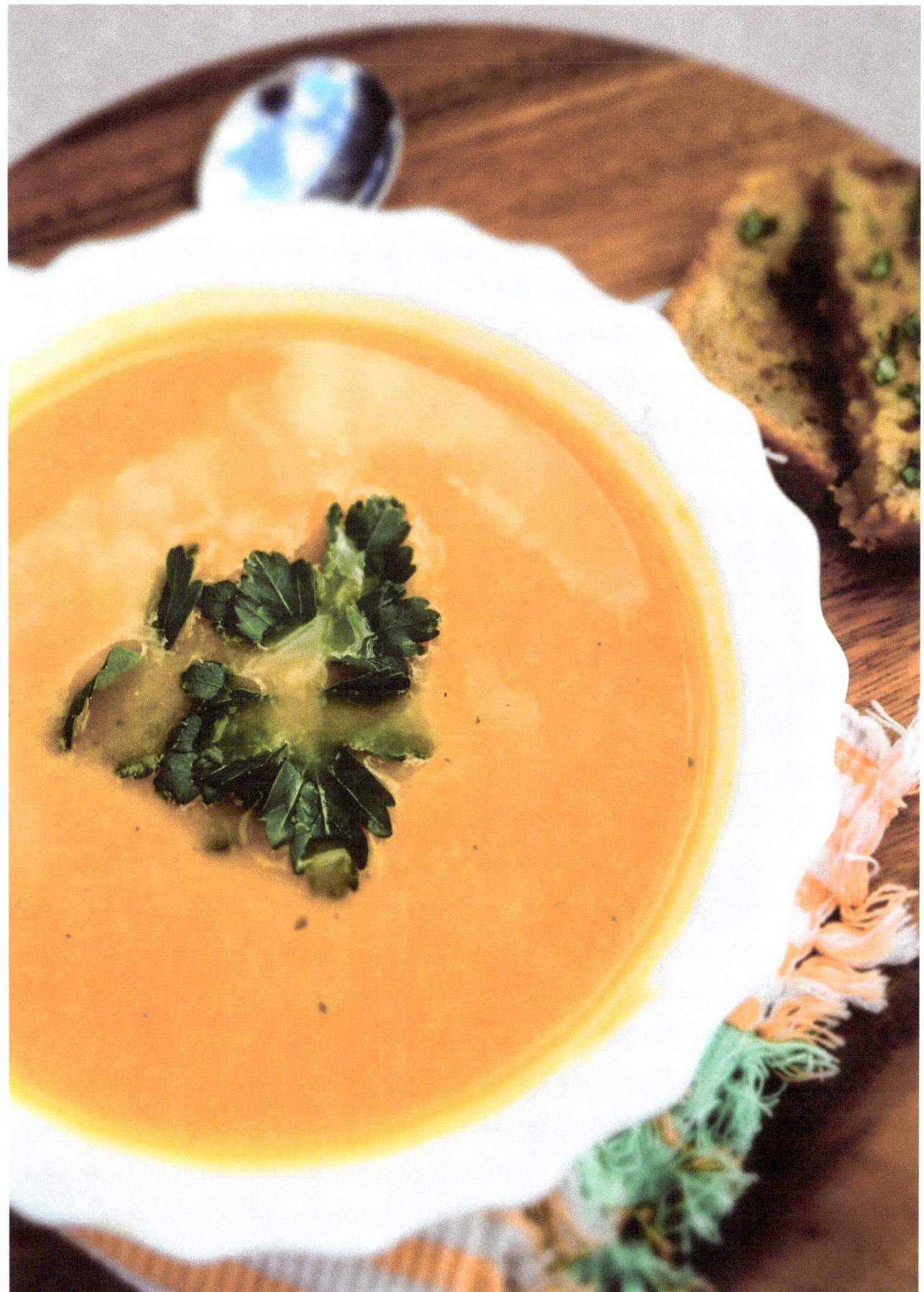

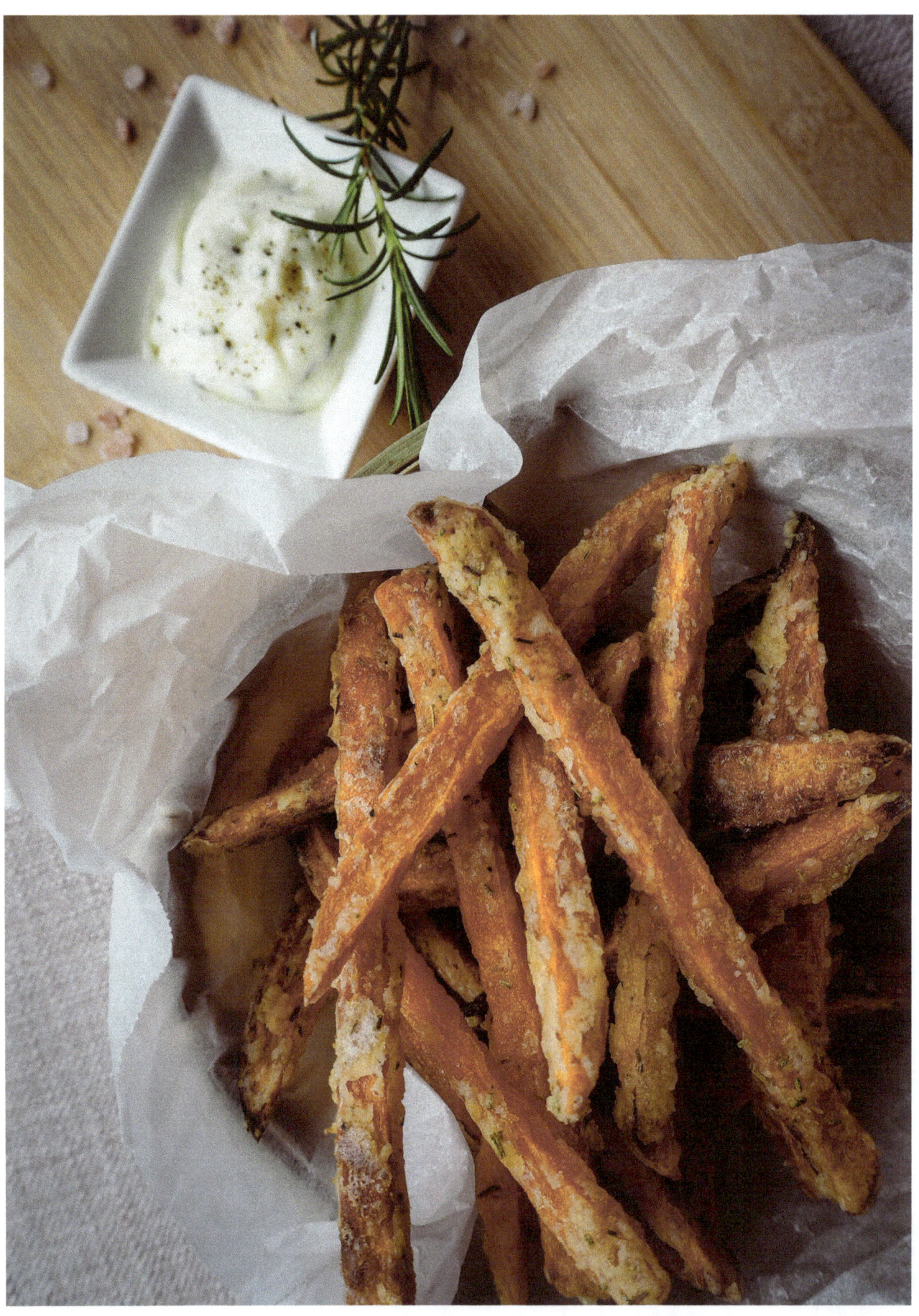

Baked Garlic & Rosemary Sweet Potato Chips

Serves 2-3 people

Fancy eating chips at home that feel and taste as if they have been deep-fried, but are super healthy and super easy to make? My baked sweet potato chips are delightfully crunchy on the outside, yet soft on the inside. You will be surprised at how tasty they are — and not a deep fryer in sight!

1 medium to large orange sweet potato
4 heaped tablespoons tapioca starch or arrowroot starch
1 - 1 ½ teaspoons salt
Garlic-infused olive oil and olive oil mix
½ teaspoon dried rosemary or 2 sprigs fresh rosemary

Peel and cut the sweet potato into 1 cm julienne pieces. In a large bowl, soak the sweet potato pieces in some iced or very cold water for roughly 1 hour.

Preheat the oven to 190°c and line a baking tray. Fill a large zip lock bag with the sweet potato pieces, salt, tapioca starch and rosemary. Seal with some air in the bag and toss back and forth to coat evenly. Drizzle garlic-infused olive oil and olive oil over the chips in the bag. Seal again and toss till evenly coated so that every piece is sufficiently battered.

Spread the chips out evenly on the lined baking tray, drizzle them with a little olive oil and bake for 40 minutes. Halfway through the baking, turn them over using a pair of tongs, to ensure even browning and crispening. If the chips need a little more time to crisp up, increase the oven temperature to 200°c and bake for another 5 minutes.

Once the chips are cooked and the batter around them is crispy, remove them from the oven and serve immediately.

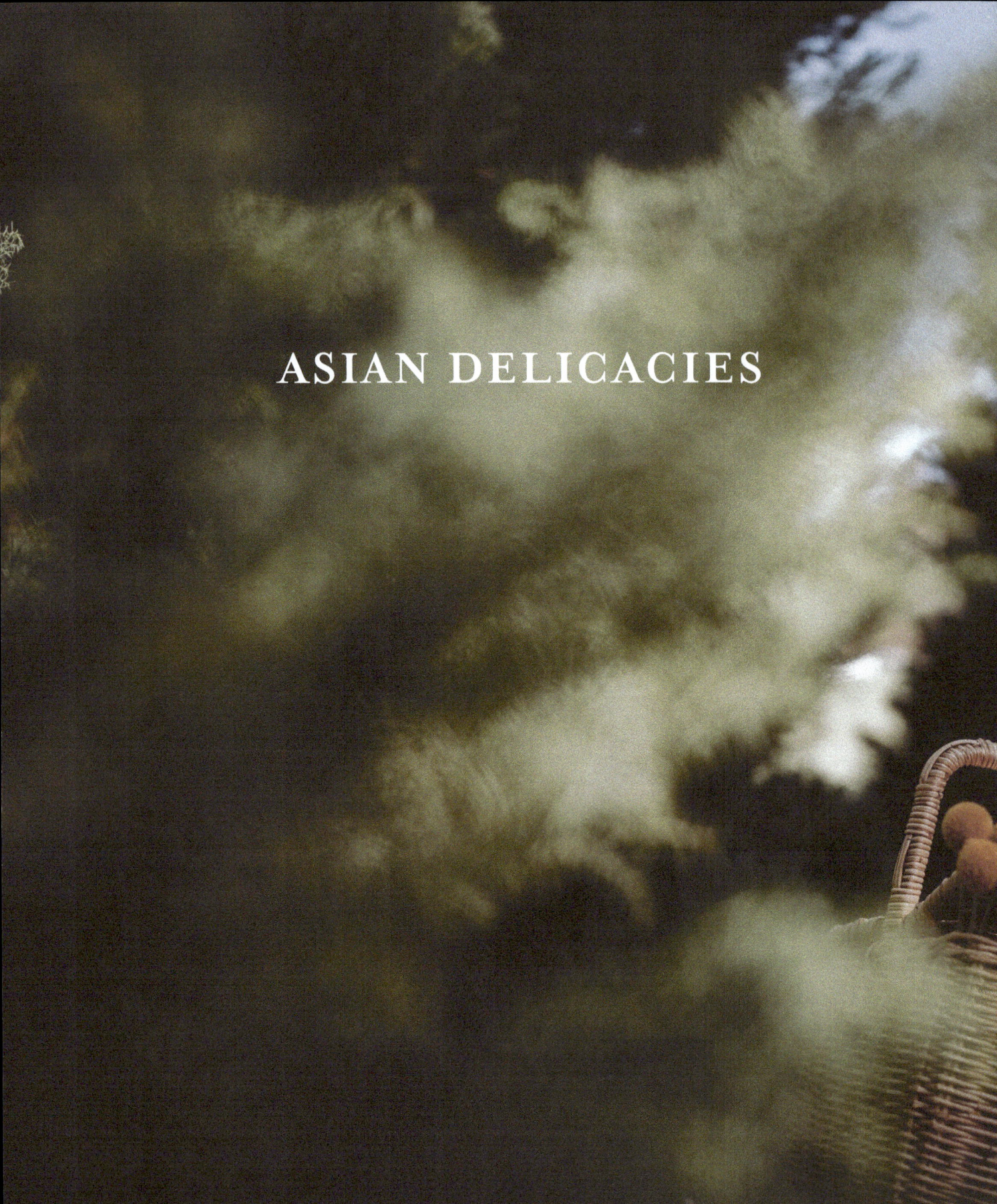
ASIAN DELICACIES

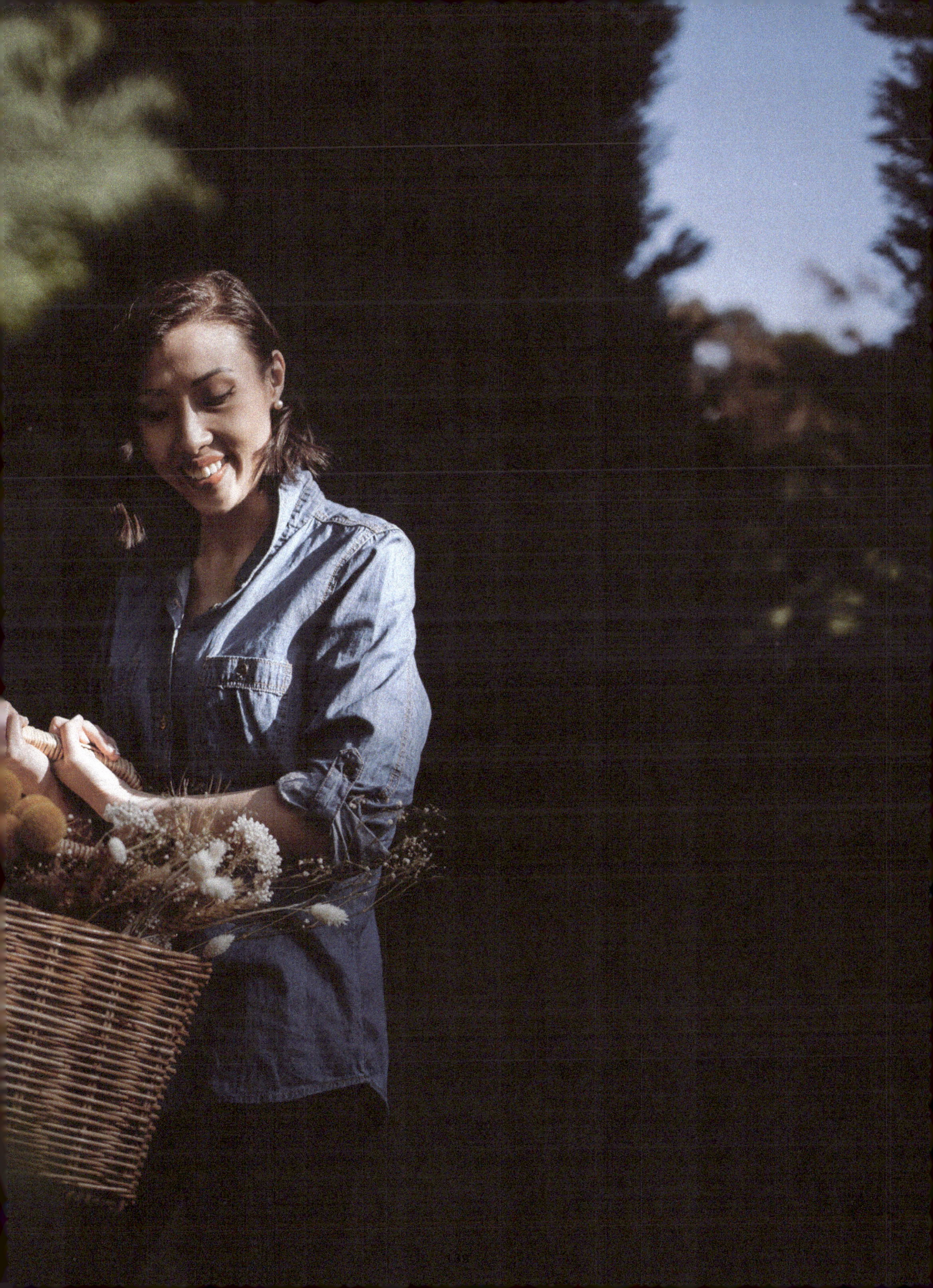

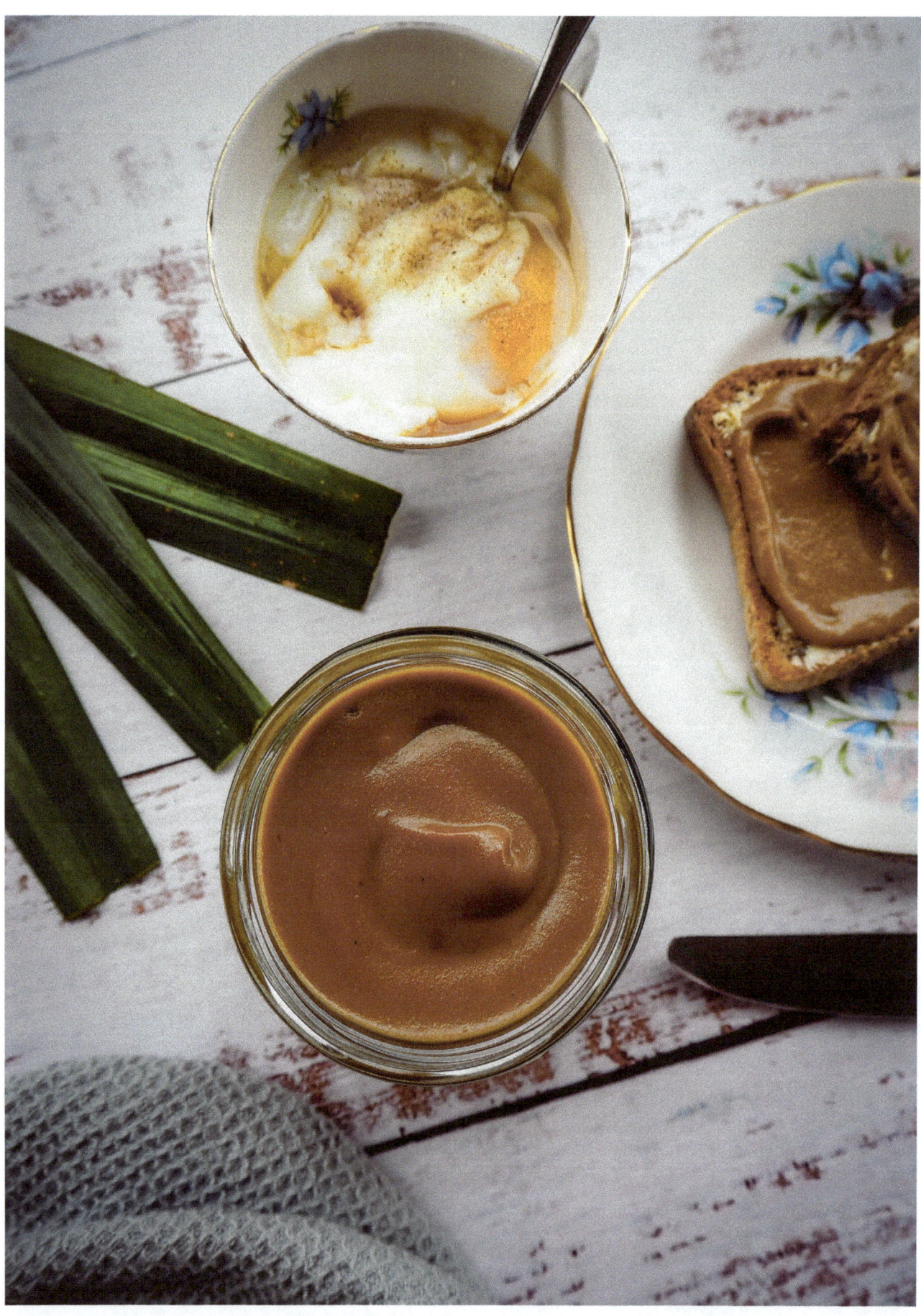

Kaya

Makes 2 medium-sized jars or 3 small jars

Kaya is famously known throughout South East Asia and is one of the staple condiments to have in many households and food establishments. It is usually served for breakfast on buttered toast with a side of soft-boiled eggs and coffee, or eaten as a snack in the form of a sweet filling encased in puff pastry or soft bao buns. Kaya is a smooth coconut egg jam; infused with the flavour and aroma of pandan and unrefined palm sugar, known as Gula Melaka, giving it its unique taste profile. Kaya is commonly sold in two different forms; a green-coloured or a brown-coloured jam. Some are sweetened with sugar, honey and a hint of ginger, while others are sweetened with refined sugar and pandan essence, with artificial green food colouring added. This recipe uses authentic unrefined palm sugar and fresh pandan leaves while staying true to its natural colour. I love mine with a hint of ginger which is influenced by my Hainanese heritage. If you haven't tried this creamy spread yet, you are guaranteed to love it!

4 jumbo or 5 regular free-range eggs
190 g unrefined palm sugar (authentic Gula Melaka) or coconut sugar
½ cup organic coconut cream
¾ cup organic coconut milk
3 pandan leaves, washed and tied in a knot
2 teaspoons tapioca starch or arrowroot starch mixed with 2 teaspoons of water
1 tablespoon vegan butter for added gloss (optional)
1 small knob of fresh thinly sliced ginger for added flavour (optional)

In a mixing bowl, whisk together the eggs, coconut milk and coconut cream until combined. Pour the mixture through a sieve into a wide rimmed pan or large saucepan, to remove any egg bits.

Grate the hardened palm sugar and add it into the mixture (or if using coconut sugar, add together in the first step). Make small incisions on the edges of the pandan leaves to let the flavour infuse into the kaya jam and add in the knotted pandan leaves and/or fresh slices of ginger into the coconut mixture.

On low heat, continuously stir with a wooden spoon for about 15-20 minutes from commencement. It is normal for the jam to become lumpy from the cooked eggs so don't be concerned as this will become smooth once it is blended later on.

Add in the vegan butter (optional) and the arrowroot slurry, then stir well to combine until thickened. Cook for another 3-4 minutes. Remove the pan from the stove to allow it to cool down for about 10 minutes. Once cooled, remove the pandan leaves and ginger pieces. Pour the kaya into a food processor or blender and blend until the jam is smooth and glossy.

RECIPE NOTES

The kaya jam should last for 2 weeks in the fridge.

It is crucial that the kaya is not overcooked on the stove, as it will not be as smooth or glossy after it is blended. Once it splits, you have overcooked it.

Pandan Sponge Cake

Makes 8-10 slices

Growing up in Malaysia, pandan-flavoured sponge cake was one of my favourite sweet treats to have from the Chinese grocery store. Pandan leaves, otherwise known as Screwpine leaves, are popular in flavouring savoury and sweet dishes in South East Asia. Some say it is an equivalent flavouring extract to vanilla. This sponge cake is light, moist and fluffy, and exudes the aromas and nuances of pandan throughout — all without artificial flavours or colours.

4 free-range eggs, separated
½ cup maple sugar
¼ cup brown rice flour (40 g), sifted twice
⅔ cup tapioca starch (80 g), sifted twice
2 teaspoons pure vanilla extract
1 teaspoon apple cider vinegar
½ teaspoon salt
30 ml organic extra virgin coconut oil, melted
40 ml unsweetened almond milk
8 pandan leaves, washed and cut
½ to 1 teaspoon 100% natural green food colouring

Preheat the oven to 170°c and lightly grease the sides of an 18-20cm round removable-base cake tin (do not grease the base as this will affect the texture of base). Line the base of the baking tin with baking paper and set aside.

Wash and cut the pandan leaves into thick strips and place in a food processor, together with 60 ml of unsweetened almond milk (it will increase in volume to 75 ml, but the remainder can be frozen for future use). You can also use a stick mixer or equivalent equipment to blend until finely blended. Pour the blended leaves and milk mix into a sieve and press out as much of the pandan extract as possible. Set aside 40 ml of the pandan-infused almond milk and add in ½ teaspoon of natural green food colouring powder (I use Summer Hill Pantry's Fruit Sparkles 100% natural food colouring), stirring to combine. You can increase it to 1 teaspoon if desired.

Sift the brown rice flour and tapioca starch together twice and set aside. Measure out 30 ml of coconut oil and set aside. Separate the egg yolks and egg whites.

In a mixing bowl, beat the egg whites and apple cider vinegar together until soft peaks form. Slowly incorporate the maple sugar while continuously beating the egg whites. Once all the sugar is incorporated, beat the mixture until stiff peaks form. Add in the egg yolks, using a whisk to mix together. Add in the sifted flour and salt in increments while whisking gently in a folding action.

Once mixed well, add in the coconut oil, pandan-infused almond milk and vanilla extract and gently fold with the whisk, then change to a spatula to finish combining it all together.

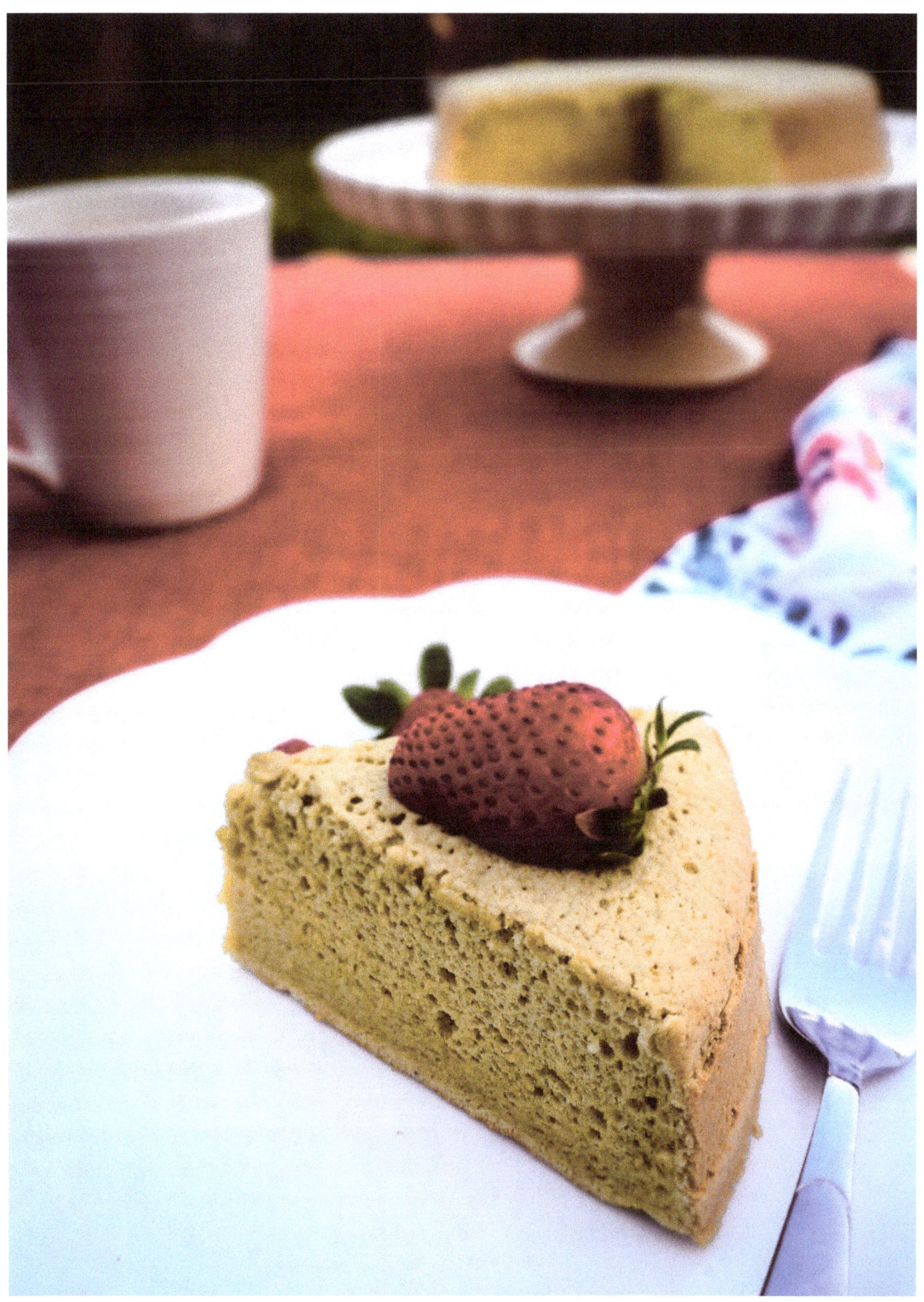

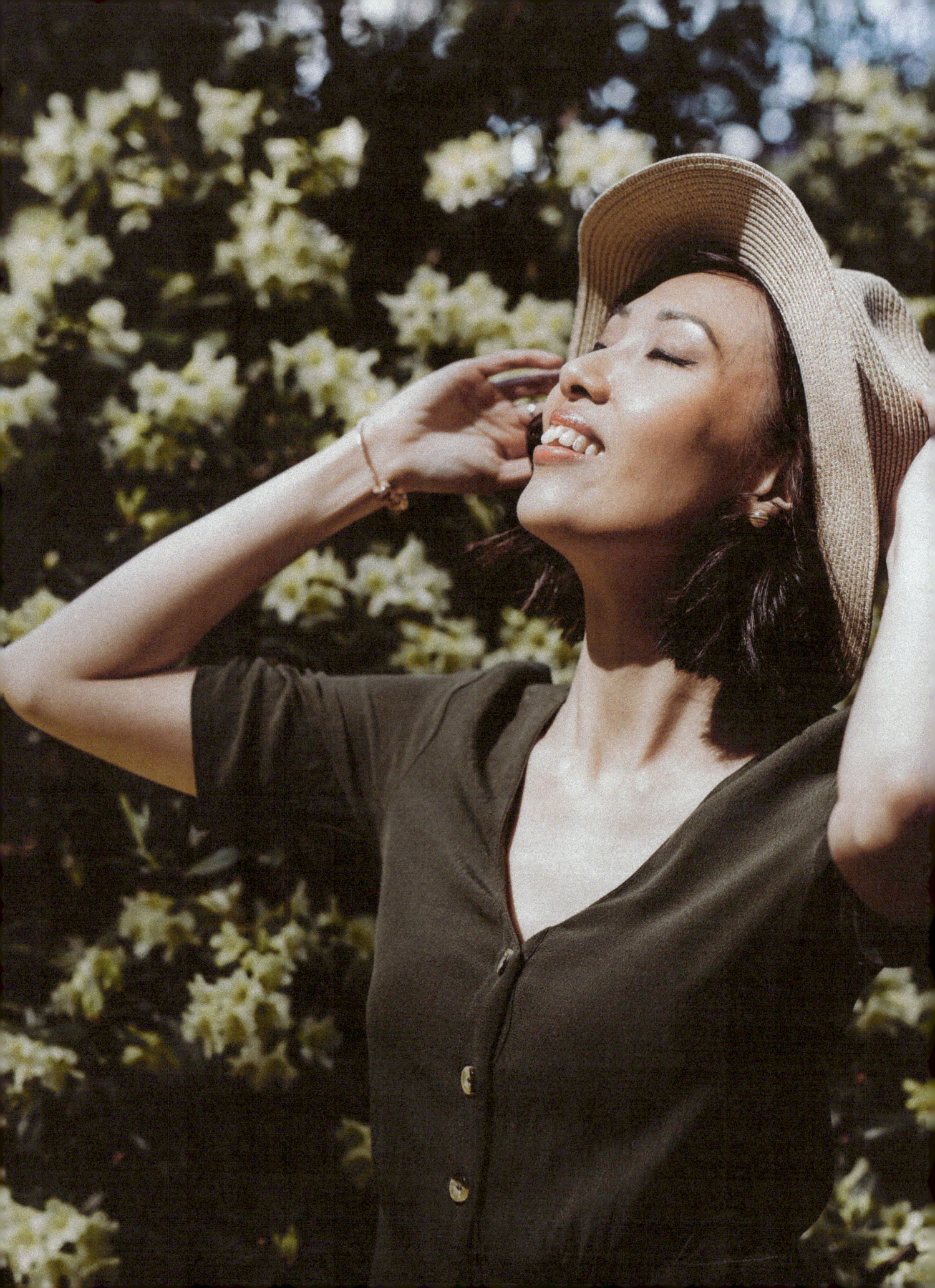

Pandan Sponge Cake Continued —

Spoon the batter into the cake tin, gently tapping the tin twice to remove any air bubbles. Bake for 25-30 minutes or until a skewer inserted in the centre of the cake comes out clean.

Let the cake cool in the tin for 5 minutes, then remove the base and lift the baking paper, carrying the cake onto a wire rack to cool completely before cutting. Do not let the cake sit in the tin for longer than 10 minutes, or the residual heat will cook the base, resulting in a rubbery texture.

RECIPE NOTES

Making this cake requires you to work fast, so measure and prepare all the ingredients first before the egg whites are whipped up. The goal is for the beaten egg whites to maintain their initial stiff peaks, resulting in a sponge that will rise well.

It is crucial to use a whisk to mix the batter up until the spatula is used at the end, as this helps the ingredients to combine well without over-stirring. Over-stirring will result in a sponge that is dense and flat, rather than light and fluffy.

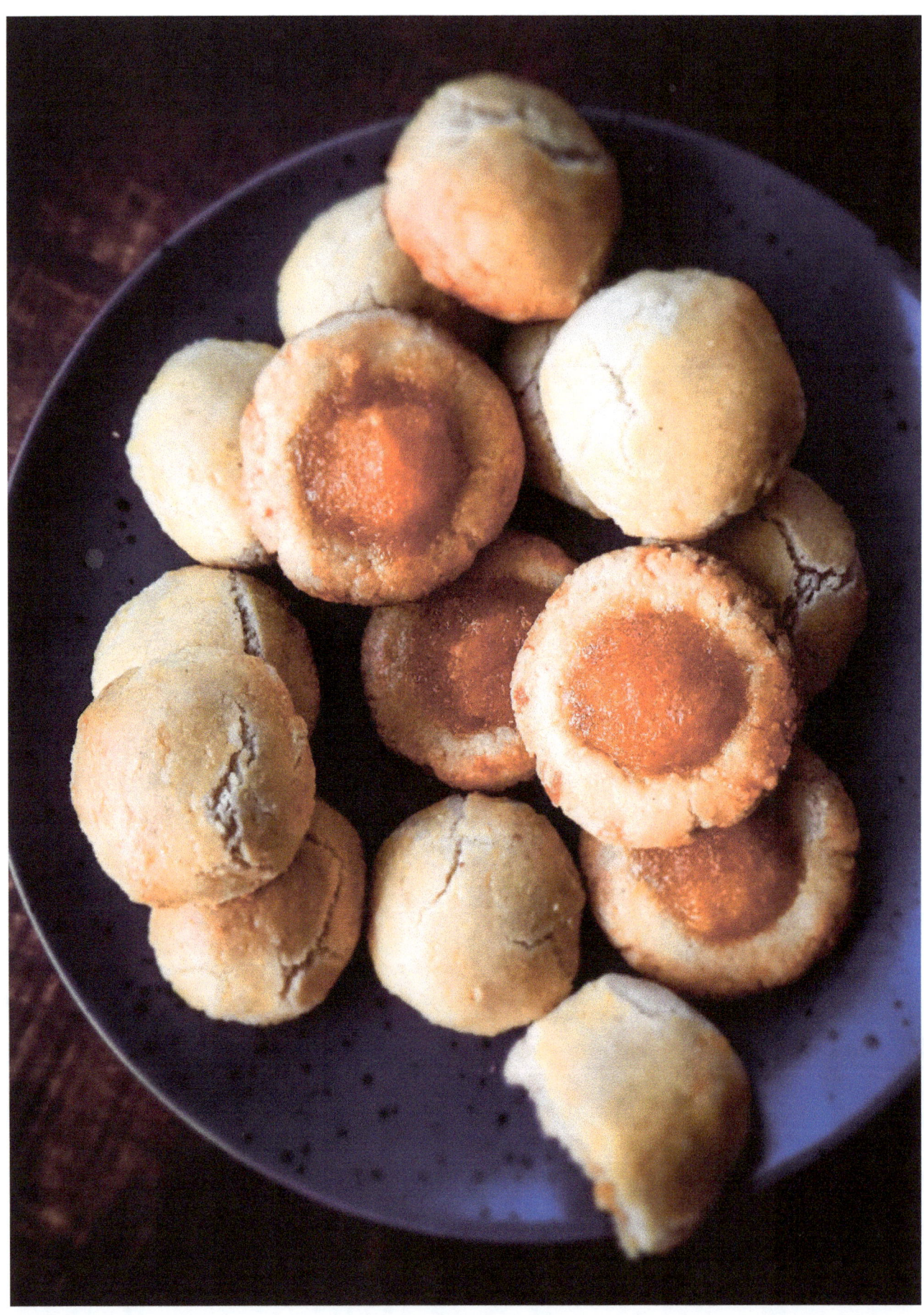

Pineapple Tarts

*Makes 32 encased tarts or
20 encased and 13 open tarts*

Pineapple tarts are a Chinese New Year treat and popularly sold at Chinese grocery stores leading up to the event. The sweet and sticky pineapple jam is enveloped by crumbly and buttery pastry, making every bite a melting moment. Whether you make them rolled up or like jam drops, they make for an enticing treat — it's hard to stop at just one!

PINEAPPLE JAM
MAKES ¾ - 1 CUP
1 whole ripe organic pineapple
½ cup pure maple syrup
1 tablespoon coconut sugar (optional - only add in if the pineapple is lacking in sweetness)
1 cinnamon quill
½ star anise
2 cloves
¼ teaspoon salt

BISCUIT PASTRY
2 cups blanched almond flour
⅔ cup tapioca starch
⅓ cup millet flour or sorghum flour
½ teaspoon pure vanilla extract
⅓ cup organic extra virgin coconut oil, melted
¼ cup pure maple syrup
Water (1-2 teaspoons to bind if mixture is dry)
¼ teaspoon salt

EGG WASH
1 egg yolk
1 tablespoon unsweetened almond milk

PINEAPPLE JAM
Cut the pineapple and blend the pieces until you have a pureed consistency. Pour the pureed pineapple through a sieve or muslin cloth to strain the excess juice (do not drain all the juice as the jam will be too dry).

Pour the strained pineapple puree into a small saucepan and add the maple syrup, cinnamon quill, star anise, cloves and salt.

Bring the mixture to a boil, then lower to a simmer for 40 minutes, stirring frequently. Once the jam has cooled, refrigerate for a few hours or better still, overnight.

BISCUIT PASTRY & ASSEMBLING
In a mixing bowl, whisk the almond flour and tapioca starch together, then add in the remaining ingredients and mix until a dough forms. If the mixture is too dry, add in a little water to bind it all together. Wrap the dough in cling wrap and refrigerate for 15-20 minutes to rest.

Preheat the oven to 180°c and line two baking trays. Once the dough is out of the fridge, spoon roughly 1 tablespoon of dough and flatten it in your palm. Add 1 teaspoon of the pineapple filling into the centre of the dough then fold the pastry over on all sides and pinch to seal the edges. This process should make a round shape. Repeat this process until all the dough is used up. If you prefer, you can make open pineapple tarts instead, by flattening the dough slightly in your palm and spooning a teaspoon-sized dollop of pineapple jam in the middle of the dough. Once you have used all the dough, you should have a little bit of leftover pineapple filling.

Place the pineapple tarts onto the lined baking trays and brush each tart with the egg wash. Bake for 10-20 minutes until they appear golden brown. Once out of the oven, let the tarts cool on a wire rack and store in an airtight container.

Baked Egg Tarts

*Makes 8 (with 9.5 cm tart tins) or
12 (with a standard cupcake mould tin)*

Egg tarts are another well-loved classic Chinese delight that you would typically see served up at 'yum cha'* or at Chinese street vendors and cafes. Whether they come in buttery shortcrust pastry cases or flaky puff pastry shells, egg tarts have evolved into several different varieties over time, like many dishes developed in the past. These little wonders consist of a smooth and sweet vanilla egg custard, nestled in a crumbly but sturdy shortcrust pastry, with a sprinkling of cinnamon on top. Put the kettle on because these egg tarts are waiting to be tasted.

SHORTCRUST PASTRY
Refer to Slice and Tart Base — Option 2 on page 86

EGG CUSTARD
1 ¼ cups unsweetened almond milk
4 free-range eggs
2 teaspoons pure vanilla extract
⅓ cup maple sugar
⅛ teaspoon salt

OPTIONAL
Sprinkle a hint of cinnamon on the freshly baked egg tarts

Preheat the oven to 190°C and grease a 12-mould standard cupcake tin. Make the shortcrust pastry by referring to the Slice and Tart Base — Option 2 recipe on page 86. Once the dough has rested in the fridge for 1 hour, take it out and place on a generously floured board. Dust the dough lightly with some gluten-free flour, then roll it out until it is 3 mm thick.

Using a 10 cm biscuit cutter, cut circles in the dough and place each into the cupcake moulds. You will need to re-group the dough to flatten out and cut more circles until all 12 cupcake moulds are filled. Gently ease the cut-out dough into the cupcake moulds, making sure all sides are covered and at an even thickness.

Alternatively, if the dough is a little on the soft side once it is out of the fridge (this can depend on the type of butter or oil you use), simply dust the dough with some gluten-free flour, knead it a little and then divide the dough into 12 even-sized balls. Place each ball in each of the 12 cupcake moulds and begin to press them evenly into the moulds, roughly 3 mm in thickness on all sides and the bottom. This process is slightly more labour-intensive, but the results will be the same.

Once all the moulds are filled, use a fork to make holes throughout the bases before placing them in the oven to bake. Blind bake the tarts for 15 minutes. Once the tart shells are out of the oven, reduce the oven temperature to 150°C.

While the tart shells are cooling, prepare the egg custard filling. In a saucepan, heat up the almond milk and vanilla extract until just simmering.

In a mixing bowl, whisk the eggs and maple sugar together. Slowly pour in the hot milk mixture, whisking continuously to avoid scrambling the eggs with the heat. Pour the custard mixture through a fine sieve into a glass jug, ensuring it is as smooth as possible.

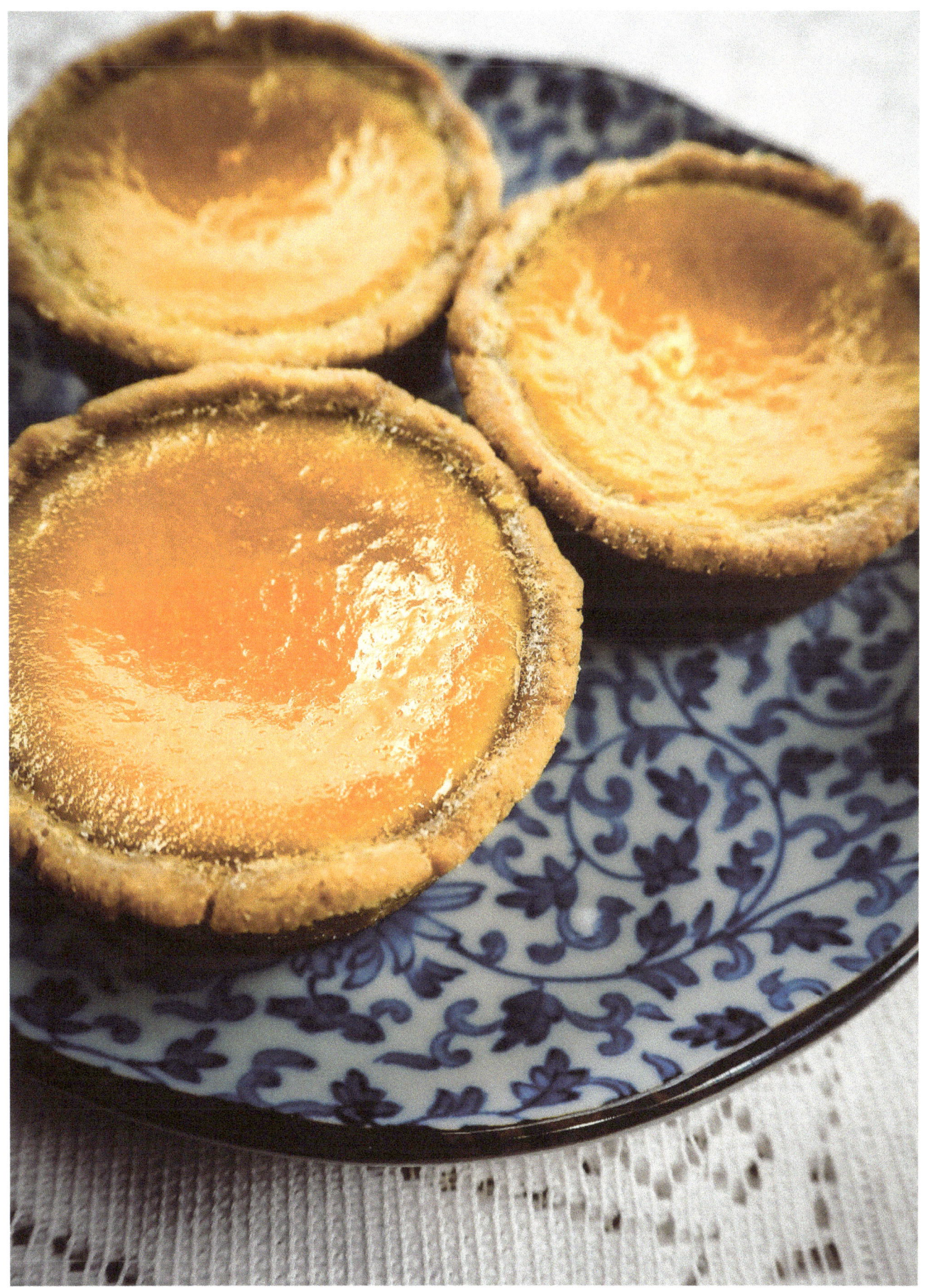

Baked Egg Tarts Continued —

Carefully pour the egg custard mixture into the tart shells, filling it up as close as possible to the top. If there are bubbles on the surface, use a teaspoon to remove them. Place the egg tarts in the oven and bake for 30 minutes or until the egg custard is just set.

You must watch the egg tarts closely because if the custard puffs up too much during baking, it will shrink down substantially once it is cooled. This shrinking will result in an egg custard that is not smooth and level. If the custard starts to puff up in the oven, reduce the oven temperature to 140°c and leave the oven door slightly ajar for 2-3 minutes. Then, close the door and continue baking the egg tarts at 140°c until just set, which could take another 10-15 minutes.

Once the egg custard has just set, turn the oven off and open the oven door, leaving the egg tarts to begin cooling down in the oven for about 10 minutes, before removing them out of the oven to cool even further. This strategy will ensure the egg custard filling does not shrink too quickly with the drastic temperature change. Serve warm.

RECIPE NOTES

The egg tarts can be stored in an airtight container in the fridge for up to 3 days.

To reheat the egg tarts, place in the oven for 10 minutes at 150°c.

*'Yum Cha' literally means 'drink tea', and refers to the experience of drinking tea and eating 'dim sum', which is a style of Chinese cuisine in which bite-sized portions of food are served on small plates or in small steamer baskets.

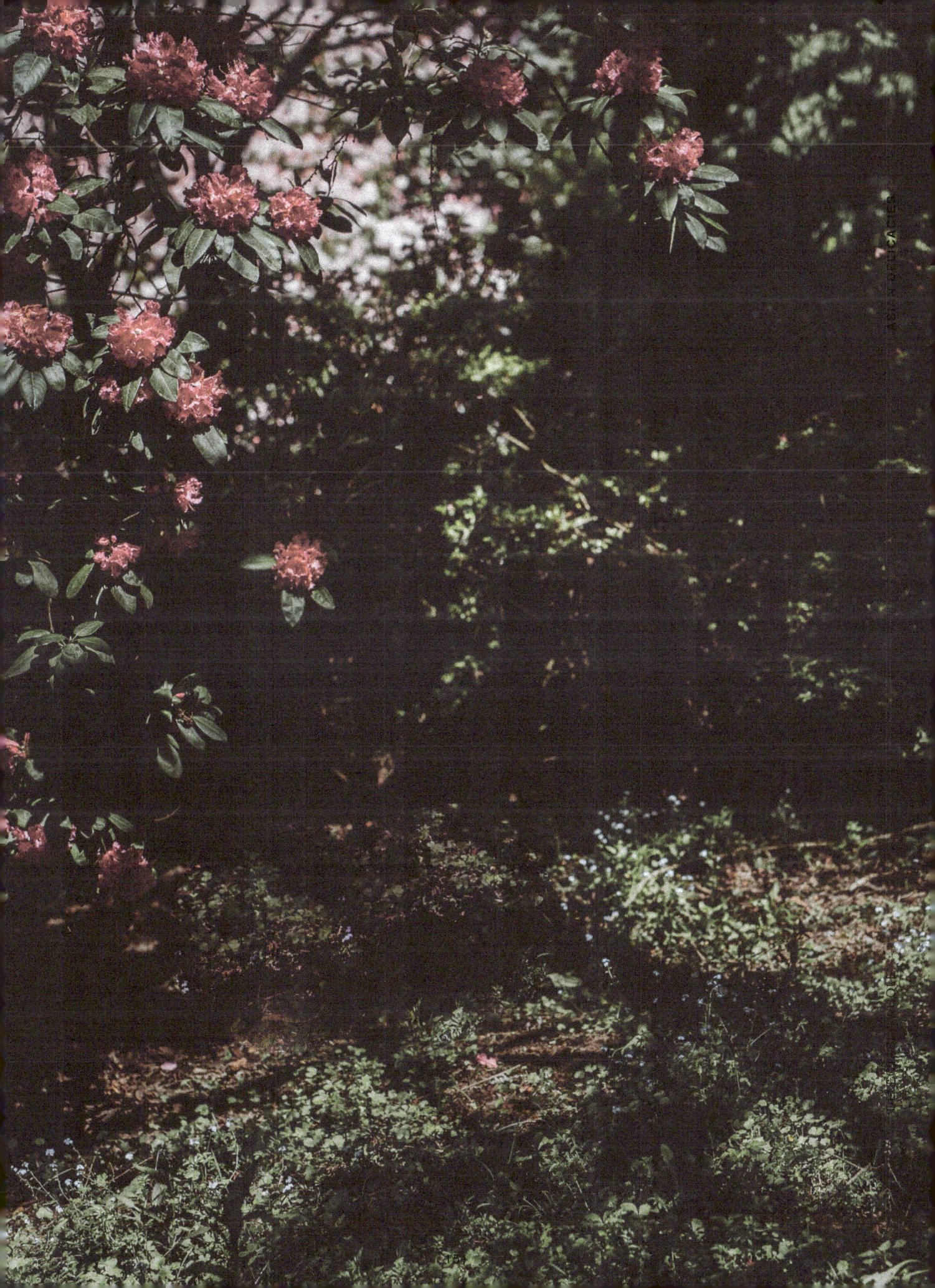

REFERENCES

ASEA 2016, *Redox Signaling*, viewed 15 February 2020, <https://aseaglobal.com/science/redoxsignaling/>.

Barnes, Whitney 2018, *All About Starches,* Bob's Red Mill Natural Foods, viewed 13 February 2020, <https://www.bobsredmill.com/blog/featured-articles/all-about-starches/>.

Buy Organics Online 2020, *Maple Sugar*, viewed 13 February 2020, <https://www.buyorganicsonline.com.au/maple-sugar/>.

Cara 2013, *Guide to Gluten-Free Flours,* Fork & Beans, viewed 13 February 2020, <https://www.forkandbeans.com/2013/12/30/guide-gluten-free-flours/ >.

Christine 2019, *5 Alternatives to Xantham Gum and Guar Gum in Gluten-Free Baking,* Zest for Baking, viewed 13 February 2020, <https://zestforbaking.com/5-alternatives-to-xanthan-gum-and-guar-gum-in-gluten-free-baking>.

Covington, Linnea 2020, *What is Tiger Nut Flour?,* The Spruce Eats, viewed 13 February 2020, <https://www.thespruceeats.com/what-is-tigernut-flour-4771200>.

DiValentino, Ariana 2019, *11 Things You can Cook With Apple Cider Vinegar,* INSIDER, viewed 13 February 2020, <https://www.insider.com/things-you-can-make-with-apple-cider-vinegar-2019-5>.

Dr. Axe 2020, *Nutrition*, viewed 13 February 2020, <https://draxe.com/nutrition/>.

Gluten-Free Alchemist 2020, *What is Gluten-Free Flour? A Guide to the Gluten-Free Flour Mix*, viewed 13 February 2020, <https://www.glutenfreealchemist.com/p-gluten-free-flours-and-flour-blends/>.

Gruss, Teri 2018, *Gluten-Free Flour and Starch Glossary,* The Spruce Eats, viewed 13 February 2020, <https://www.thespruceeats.com/gluten-free-flour-and-starch-glossary-1451205>.

Hoover, Michelle 2018, *The Ultimate Guide to Tigernut Flour,* Unbound Wellness, viewed 13 February 2020, <https://unboundwellness.com/the-ultimate-guide-to-tigernut-flour/>.

Monash University 2019, *High and Low FODMAP Foods*, viewed 13 February 2020, <https://www.monashfodmap.com/about-fodmap-and-ibs/high-and-low-fodmap-foods/>.

Otto's Naturals 2020, *Cassava Flour,* viewed 13 February 2020, <https://www.ottosnaturals.com/>.

Outback Harvest Teff Team 2019, *Our Top Tips for Cooking With Teff Flour*, viewed 13 February 2020, <https://outbackharvest.com.au/blogs/top-tips-for-cooking-with-teff-flour>.

Schar 2020, *An In-Depth Guide to 12 Popular Gluten-Free Flours*, viewed 13 February 2020, <https://www.schaer.com/en-us/a/gluten-free-flours>.

Scott, Alana 2015, *What Nuts are Low FODMAP?,* A Little Bit Yummy, viewed 13 February 2020, <https://alittlebityummy.com/what-nuts-are-low-fodmap/>.

Trang 2020, *Rice Flour vs Glutinous Rice Flour - What are the Differences?',* RunAwayRice, viewed 13 February 2020, <https://runawayrice.com/cooking-basics/rice-flour-vs-glutinous-rice-flour-what-are-the-differences/>.

Uncle Toby's 2020, *Australian Oats - What is an Oat?*, viewed 13 February 2020, <https://www.uncletobys.com.au/australian-oats/all-about-oats/what-is-an-oat>.

Zimberoff, Larissa 2016, *Master of Bun: Sift Through Our Guide to All the Flour Varieties You'll Ever Need,* Tasting Table, viewed 13 February 2020, <https://www.tastingtable.com/cook/national/flour-types-varieties-guide-baking-gluten-free-wheat-bread-guide>.

FOOTNOTES

*Both the ASEA Redox drinking water and RENU28 gel activate our body's immune system to combat disease and inflammation by supplying our bodies with Redox Signalling Molecules that our cells already naturally produce (however, diminish due to aging and disease).

ASEA helps provide the groundwork for identifying, repairing, replenishing and replacing damaged cells caused by the body's inability to effectively detoxify itself. For more information, check out these websites:

https://aseascience.com/

https://aseaglobal.com/

Please be aware that cooking times may vary for each recipe, depending on the type of oven used.

All teaspoon, tablespoon and cup measurements used in these recipes are based on the Australian metric measuring system.

Gratitude

This cookbook from its inception to what I now hold in my hands, would not exist without the One who is my strength, motivator, helper, joy-giver and counsellor. He is the greatest inventor and master of all chefs in this world — Jesus. You held my dream, passion, gifts and abilities in Your hands and walked with me every step of the way with such patience, tenderness, love, mercy and grace to make what seemed impossible, possible. This book is dedicated to You.

My sincere gratefulness to my family — Mum, Dad, my sister Mec-Tsyn and Michael for helping make this cookbook a reality. Thank you for your time, encouragement and investment in helping it be the best version it can be and for all of your hard work, sacrifice and love.

My deepest gratitude to my 'bestie', Nartarsha for cheering me on every single day, for your investment, support, care and love. Thank you for being a willing taste-tester along with my family; sorry for all the cold meals you had to put up with so I could capture the best photo! I could not have accomplished this massive feat without you.

My heartfelt thanks to Ilana (Lani) for your creative brilliance and magnificent work in helping to transform my vision into something bigger and better than I could have ever imagined! It was such a pleasure and an honour to work with you. A huge thank you to Catherine for your impeccable skill and incredible eye in capturing the most stunning photos with such heart, passion and style. I had so much fun working with you; it was such a joy.

Special note of appreciation to Andria and Jozua for your guidance and patience in walking me through the uncharted waters of the publishing process — I am truly grateful. To my extended family and friends (both near and far) — thank you for believing in me, for your faithful encouragement and prayers, and for sharing your pearls of wisdom with me along the way.

Lastly, to the ones who have joined in with me on this culinary ride of a book, it has been a privilege to share my journey and recipes with you. I am truly humbled. Thank you for all your support!

Gold-Crested Press
Beaconsfield, Victoria 3807, Australia
Gold-Crested Press is the quality self-publishing imprint of Cardinia Ranges Publishing House enabling, through quality-guarantee and distribution, independent authors to inspire people.

Title: Delectably Whole
Copyright ©2020 by Mec-Lynn Lee
First published 2020

All rights reserved. Apart from any fair dealing for the purpose of private study, research, criticism or review, as permitted under the Copyright Act, no part may be reproduced by any process without written permission from the author. Inquiries should be addressed to Gold-Crested Press.

ISBN: 978-1-922537-00-3

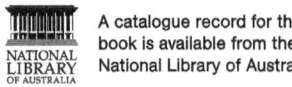

A catalogue record for this book is available from the National Library of Australia

Cover & interior book creative design by Ilana McMorran
Photography by Catherine Elise Photography
Food preparation & styling by Mec-Lynn Lee
Food photography by Mec-Lynn Lee
Food photography editing by Ilana McMorran
Editing by Mec-Tsyn Dawson
Proofreading by Mec-Tsyn Dawson and Mec-Lynn Lee

www.ingramcontent.com/pod-product-compliance
Lightning Source LLC
Chambersburg PA
CBHW051255110526
44588CB00026B/3001